Atlas of Histology for Medical Students

Atlas of Histology for Medical Students

Shilpi Gupta Dixit
MBBS MD DNB FIMSA MNAMS MAMS
Additional Professor
Department of Anatomy
All India Institute of Medical Sciences (AIIMS)
Jodhpur (Rajasthan), India

Surajit Ghatak
MBBS MD MAMS
Professor and Head
Department of Anatomy
All India Institute of Medical Sciences (AIIMS)
Jodhpur (Rajasthan), India

Foreword
Sanjeev Misra
MS MCh FRCS (Eng) FRCS (Glas) FICS FACS (USA) FAMS FNASc
Director and CEO
All India Institute of Medical Sciences (AIIMS)
Jodhpur (Rajasthan), India

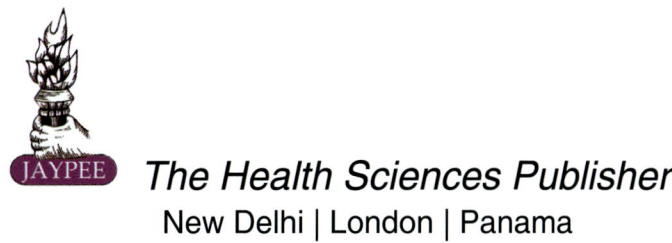

The Health Sciences Publisher
New Delhi | London | Panama

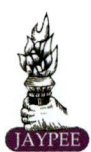
Jaypee Brothers Medical Publishers (P) Ltd

Headquarters
Jaypee Brothers Medical Publishers (P) Ltd
4838/24, Ansari Road, Daryaganj
New Delhi 110 002, India
Phone: +91-11-43574357
Fax: +91-11-43574314
Email: jaypee@jaypeebrothers.com

Overseas Offices

J.P. Medical Ltd
83 Victoria Street, London
SW1H 0HW (UK)
Phone: +44 20 3170 8910
Fax: +44 (0)20 3008 6180
Email: info@jpmedpub.com

Jaypee-Highlights Medical Publishers Inc
City of Knowledge, Bld. 235, 2nd Floor, Clayton
Panama City, Panama
Phone: +1 507-301-0496
Fax: +1 507-301-0499
Email: cservice@jphmedical.com

Jaypee Brothers Medical Publishers (P) Ltd
17/1-B Babar Road, Block-B, Shaymali
Mohammadpur, Dhaka-1207
Bangladesh
Mobile: +08801912003485
Email: jaypeedhaka@gmail.com

Jaypee Brothers Medical Publishers (P) Ltd
Bhotahity, Kathmandu
Nepal
Phone: +977-9741283608
Email: kathmandu@jaypeebrothers.com

Website: www.jaypeebrothers.com
Website: www.jaypeedigital.com

© 2018, Jaypee Brothers Medical Publishers

The views and opinions expressed in this book are solely those of the original contributor(s)/author(s) and do not necessarily represent those of editor(s) of the book.

All rights reserved. No part of this publication may be reproduced, stored or transmitted in any form or by any means, electronic, mechanical, photocopying, recording or otherwise, without the prior permission in writing of the publishers.

All brand names and product names used in this book are trade names, service marks, trademarks or registered trademarks of their respective owners. The publisher is not associated with any product or vendor mentioned in this book.

Medical knowledge and practice change constantly. This book is designed to provide accurate, authoritative information about the subject matter in question. However, readers are advised to check the most current information available on procedures included and check information from the manufacturer of each product to be administered, to verify the recommended dose, formula, method and duration of administration, adverse effects and contraindications. It is the responsibility of the practitioner to take all appropriate safety precautions. Neither the publisher nor the author(s)/editor(s) assume any liability for any injury and/or damage to persons or property arising from or related to use of material in this book.

This book is sold on the understanding that the publisher is not engaged in providing professional medical services. If such advice or services are required, the services of a competent medical professional should be sought.

Every effort has been made where necessary to contact holders of copyright to obtain permission to reproduce copyright material. If any have been inadvertently overlooked, the publisher will be pleased to make the necessary arrangements at the first opportunity. The **CD/DVD-ROM** (if any) provided in the sealed envelope with this book is complimentary and free of cost. **Not meant for sale**.

Inquiries for bulk sales may be solicited at: jaypee@jaypeebrothers.com

Atlas of Histology for Medical Students

First Edition: **2018**

ISBN: 978-93-5270-128-5

Printed at Nutech Print Services - India

Foreword

Histology forms an important part of Anatomy curriculum. Not only does it help understand the normal microscopic structure of the tissues, but it also forms the basis of histopathology.

"To diagnose the abnormal, you should be able to understand the normal."

The *Atlas of Histology for Medical Students* does precisely that. The book helps to understand and appreciate the normal tissue histology in a concise and crisp manner. Not only the photographs are clear, they also depict what is actually seen under the lens. The hand-made diagrams by the authors depict the true picture of the tissue, something that can be easily reproduced in the examinations and help in better understanding.

Writing a book is a no mean task and this Atlas is the testimony of the hard work put in by the authors. This book will not only help the undergraduates, but also postgraduate students of Anatomy and Pathology in better understanding of the subject.

Prof Sanjeev Misra
MS MCh FRCS (Eng) FRCS (Glas) FICS FACS (USA) FAMS FNASc
Director and CEO
All India Institute of Medical Sciences (AIIMS)
Jodhpur (Rajasthan), India

Preface

The learning of histology, or microanatomy, can be simple and enjoyable. This atlas grew out of a general principle of learning that, **anything is simple once you understand it**. Although teaching of medical undergraduates has now become more clinically oriented with focus on newer discoveries, but histology still remains one of the fundamental subparts of anatomy. Histology is a visual art based on the study of structures that cannot be seen. In order to study microanatomy, the major optical instrument available to the student is the light microscope. The conventional approach to teaching and learning histology has been identifying the tissues and cell by their microscopic structure. This book is an atlas containing microphotographs of all human tissues supplemented by hand-drawn diagrams of the same which can be easily reproduced by the students. This will be of immense value to undergraduates and postgraduates in anatomy as well as pathology. This book will be helpful for immediate identification and reproducibility of the diagrams as is required in examinations.

Keeping in mind the dictum "A picture is worth a thousand words", we have supplied each plate of pictures with salient identification features unique to the tissue or the organ. The atlas is organized to maximize ease of use and speed of learning. First, it is subdivided into 19 major chapters that correspond to 19 major areas of study—starting with cells, moving into tissues, and progressing into organ systems. Each plate has hand-drawn diagrams of the same that allows the reader to look back and forth between diagrams and microphotographs with no irksome page-turning. The important structures on each plate are labelled, and the labels are identified in the corresponding hand-drawn diagrams as well.

Lots of titles of histology are available in the market. The text is usually quite exhaustive and the diagrams are not that clear. This atlas will have microphotographs of human tissues accompanied by hand-drawn diagrams for their easy reproducibility.

Authors have been in undergraduate teaching for many years and have been examiners to various universities. They have felt that there is no single book which can be used as a ready reference for revision of identification and diagrams just before examination.

This atlas is not a comprehensive treatment of the subject matter. To make it so would have made the book very expensive. We are aware of the increasing strain on the student's pocket and intend this atlas to be affordable, which means its length must be limited. We have, nevertheless, attempted to offer a strategic sampling of key tissues and organs that should give the student a strong foundation in visual histology and have presented a large number of photomicrographs. In a sense, this atlas is as much of a science book, done in an art form.

Surajit Ghatak   **Shilpi Gupta Dixit**

Acknowledgments

There are a number of people we wish to thank who have helped create this atlas. Professor Sanjeev Misra, Director and CEO, AIIMS, Jodhpur offered the much-needed inspiration at the onset of the project. Dr Shilajit Bhattacharya, Professor of Pathology at AIIMS, Jodhpur kindly supplied us with tissues from his repository. Mr SM Nayeemuddin and Dr Pushpa Potaliya helped us with the microphotographs that appear in the atlas, and were a great pleasure to work with. Our laboratory technicians Mr Vineet Sharma, Mr Devender Rathore and Mr Shrikant Lodha were extremely helpful in many phases of materials preparation.

I, Shilpi Gupta Dixit, would like to express my thanks to my family, Dr Rakesh Dixit, Dr Anita Dixit, Ms Poonam Agarwal and Ms Ashima Gupta for their support. This book would not have been completed without the constant encouragement by my husband, Dr Abhinav Dixit. I express my gratitude to my daughter, Aadya for giving me time to complete this book.

I, Surajit Ghatak, would like to express my thanks and gratitude to my wife, Ms Manjari Ghatak and my son, Mr Abhigyaan for their constant support and encouragement.

We are also grateful to our colleagues in the Department of Anatomy, AIIMS, Jodhpur for offering some valuable suggestions. Finally, we are very grateful to the whole team of M/s Jaypee Brothers Medical Publishers (P) Ltd, who helped and guided us, Shri Jitendar P Vij (Group Chairman), Mr Ankit Vij (Group President), Ms Ritu Sharma (Director–Content Strategy), Ms Sunita Katla (PA to Group Chairman and Publishing Manager).

Contents

1. Parts of Light Microscope 1
2. Electron Microscopic Structure of Cell 2
3. Epithelium 3
4. Glands 7
5. Connective Tissue 11
6. Cartilage 15
7. Bone 19
8. Muscle 22
9. Nervous Tissue 27
10. Cardiovascular System 33
11. Lymphatic Tissue 38
12. Integumentary System 42
13. Digestive System 45
14. Respiratory System 60
15. Urinary System 64
16. Male Reproductive System 69
17. Female Reproductive System 73
18. Endocrine System 79
19. Eye 84

CHAPTER 1

Parts of Light Microscope

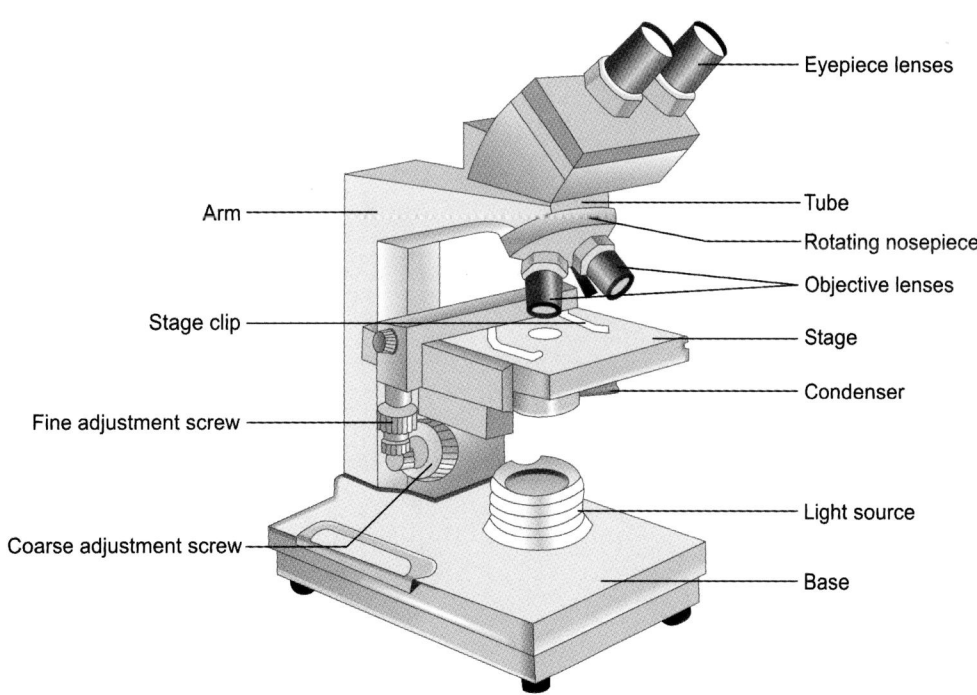

Fig. 1.1: Parts of light microscope

CHAPTER 2

Electron Microscopic Structure of Cell

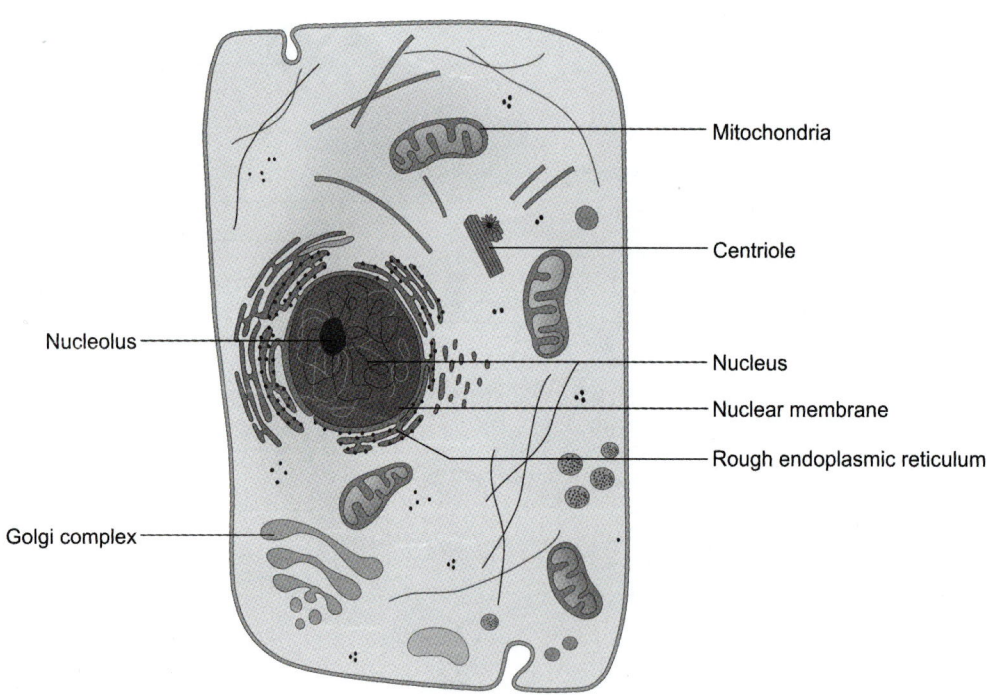

Fig. 2.1: Electron microscopic structure of cell

CHAPTER 3

Epithelium

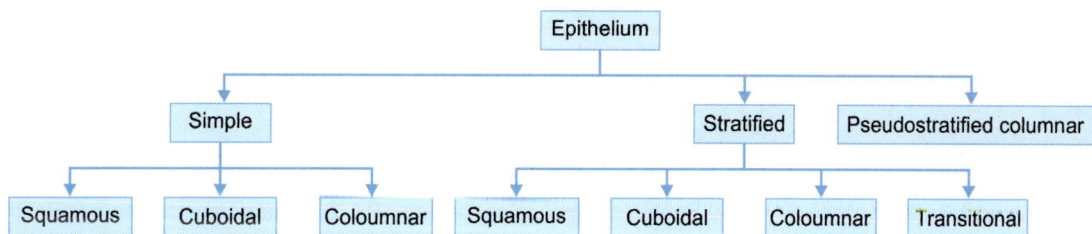

Tissue: Collection of cells organized to perform specific one or more functions.

Four basic tissue types:
- *Epithelial tissue:* Covers internal (body cavities, glands) and external surfaces of body
- *Connective tissue:* Support for other three tissues
- *Muscle tissue:* Contractile tissue for movement
- *Nervous tissue:* Receives, transmits and integrates information for control of activities of body.

Epithelium: A collection of cells, with little intercellular material.
- It covers external and internal surfaces of body.
- It may be simple or stratified.

SIMPLE EPITHELIUM

- Made up of single layer of cells.
- Several types according to cell's shape and size.
  - *Simple squamous:* Cells of epithelium are flat, having length and breadth but negligible thickness, with small, centrally placed nucleus, e.g. endothelium, Bowman's capsule, alveoli
  - *Simple cuboidal:* Cells are cubical (**L=B**), with centrally placed spherical nucleus, e.g. small ducts of exocrine glands, germinal epithelium of ovary, tubules of kidney
  - *Simple columnar:* Cells are tall in appearance (**L>B**), cytoplasm looks vacuolated due to mucinogen, and nucleus is oval in shape, e.g. stomach, small intestine, colon, gallbladder.

PSEUDOSTRATIFIED COLUMNAR EPITHELIUM

- All cells of epithelium touch the basal lamina but all of them do not reach the surface
- Nuclei are placed at different levels, giving rise to stratified look
- For example: Trachea, bronchi, ductus deferens, epididymis.

STRATIFIED EPITHELIUM

- Made up of several layers of cells
- The name of epithelium is given according to shape of cells present in the most superficial layer.
  - *Stratified squamous:* Basal cell layer consists of cuboidal or low columnar cells with mitotic activity. Intermediate layers are polygonal in shape and superficial cells are flattened, e.g. skin, oral cavity, esophagus, vagina
  - *Stratified cuboidal:* The superficial cell layer is cuboidal and rest are polyhedral in shape, e.g. large ducts of sweat and exocrine glands
  - *Stratified columnar:* The superficial layers of cells are columnar and deeper cells are polyhedral or cuboidal in shape, e.g. largest ducts of exocrine glands
  - *Transitional:* All cells are similar, being able to adjust themselves according to surface area. Basement membrane is not indented by connective tissue, e.g. bladder, ureter, urethra.

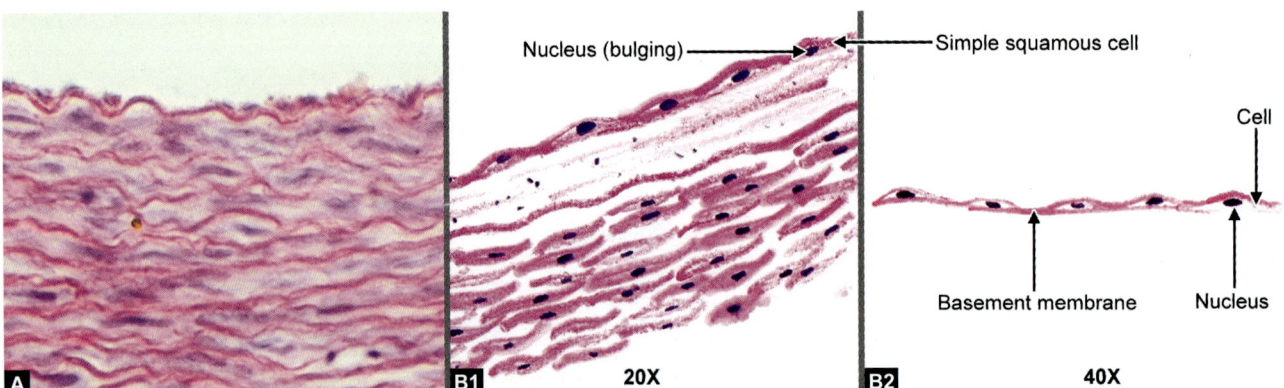

Figs 3.1A and B: (A) Microphotograph: Simple squamous epithelium; (B1, B2) Diagrammatic representation

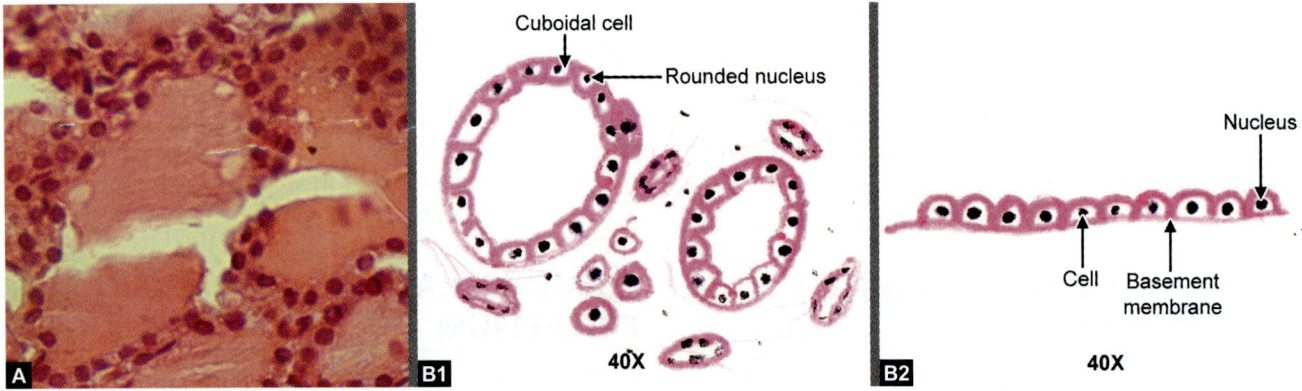

Figs 3.2A and B: (A) Microphotograph: Simple cuboidal epithelium; (B1, B2) Diagrammatic representation

Epithelium

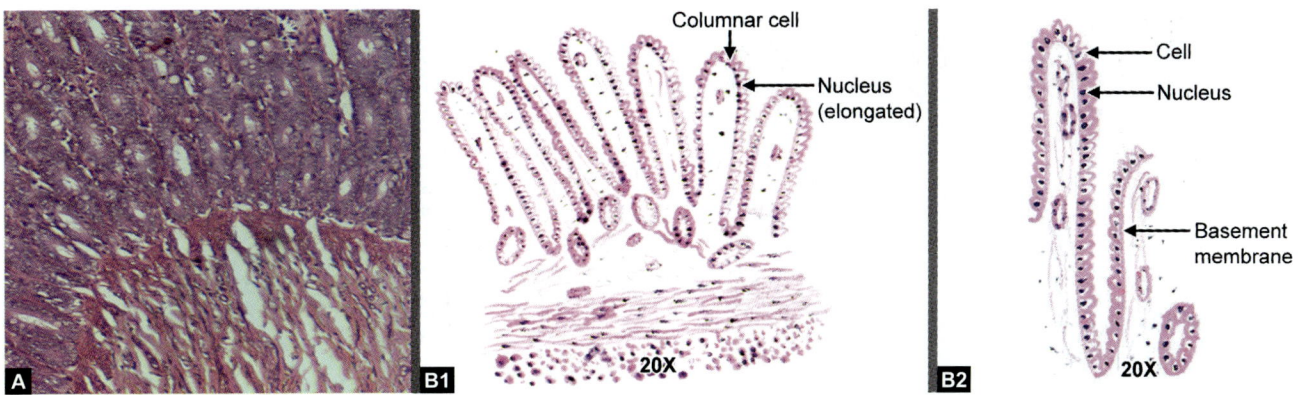

Figs 3.3A and B: (A) Microphotograph: Simple columnar epithelium; (B1, B2) Diagrammatic representation

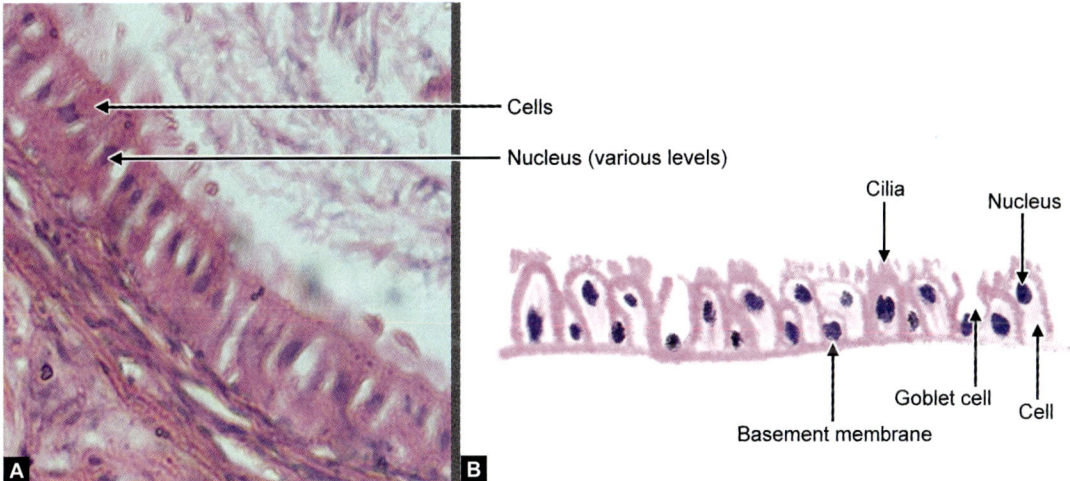

Figs 3.4A and B: (A) Microphotograph: Pseudostratified epithelium (40X); (B) Diagrammatic representation

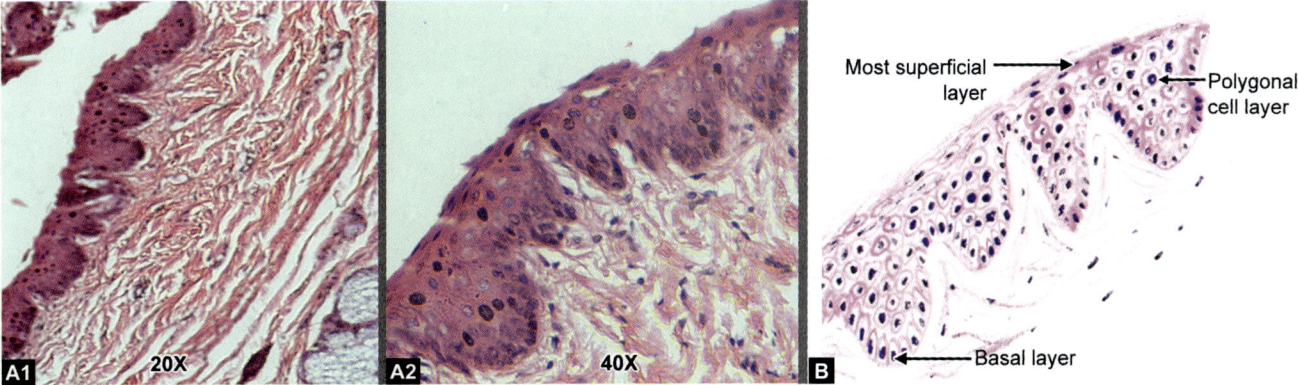

Figs 3.5A and B: (A1, A2) Microphotographs: Stratified squamous non-keratinized epithelium; (B) Diagrammatic representation

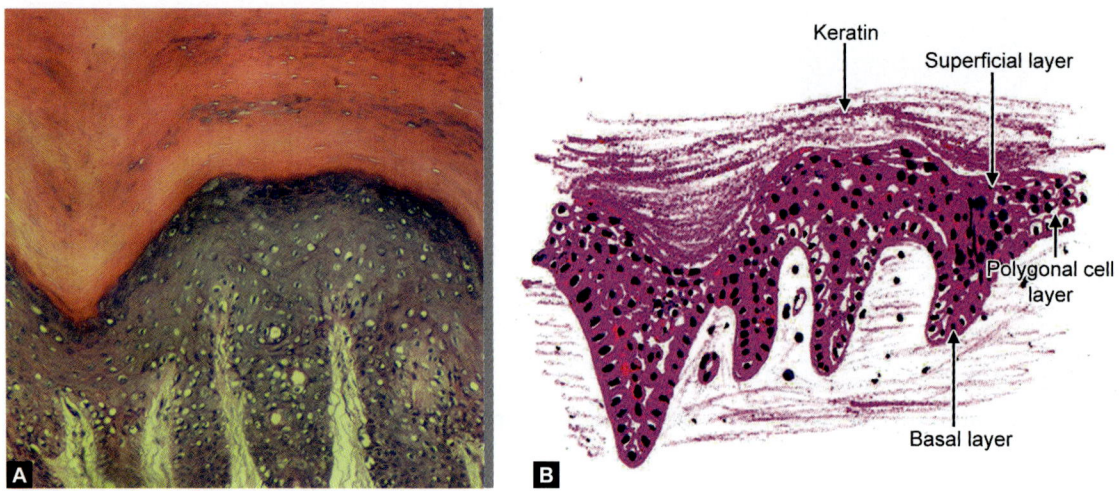

Figs 3.6A and B: (A) Microphotograph: Stratified squamous keratinized epithelium (20X); (B) Diagrammatic representation

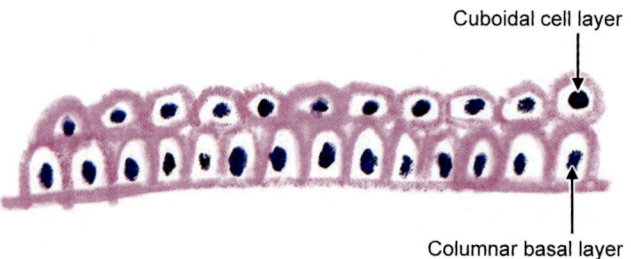

Fig. 3.7: Stratified cuboidal epithelium (40X)

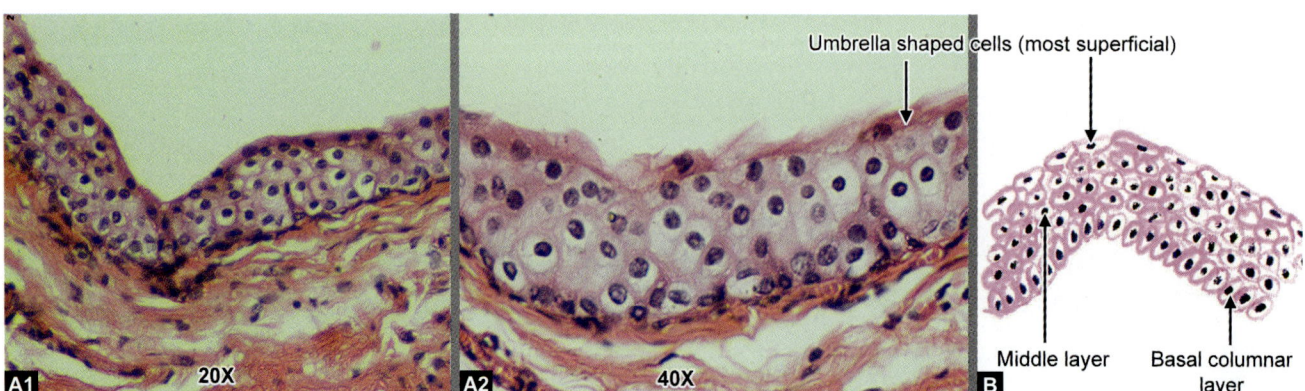

Figs 3.8A and B: (A1, A2) Microphotographs: Transitional epithelium; (B) Diagrammatic representation

CHAPTER 4

Glands

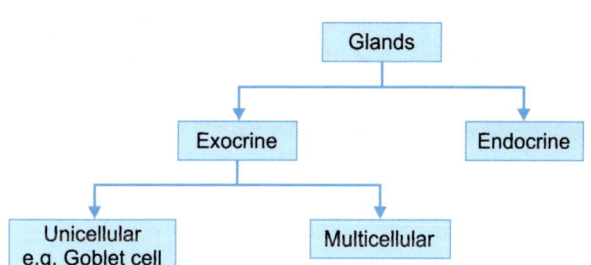

Epithelium derived secretory cells along with supporting connective tissue. Function is secretion.

Two Types of Glands

- *Exocrine:* Pour their secretion through ducts
- *Endocrine:* Pour their secretion directly into blood (capillaries).

Based on Shape of Secretory Unit

- Tubular
- Acinar
- Alveolar

Based on Number of Ducts

- Simple
- Compound

Based on Secretory Mechanism

- Merocrine
- Apocrine
- Holocrine

Based on Nature of Secretions

- Serous
- Mucous
- Mixed

8 Atlas of Histology for Medical Students

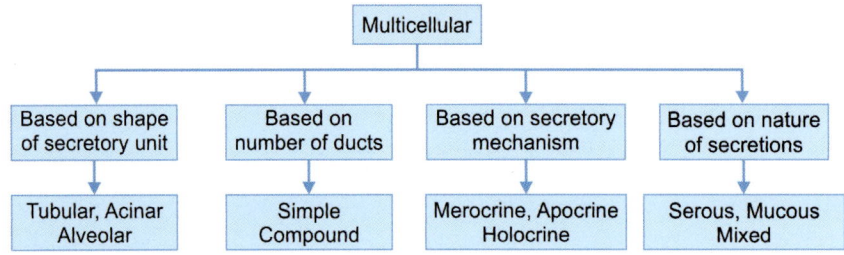

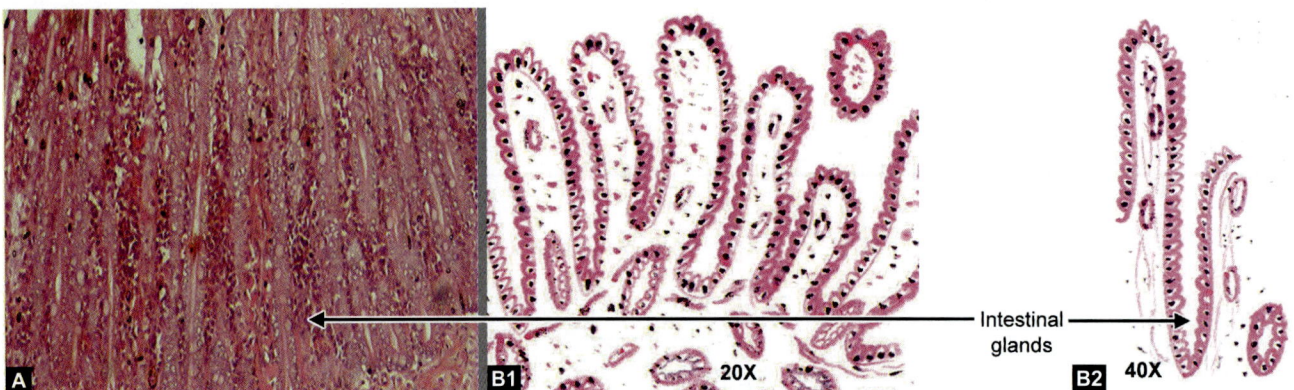

Figs 4.1A and B: (A) Microphotograph: Simple tubular gland; (B1, B2) Diagrammatic representation

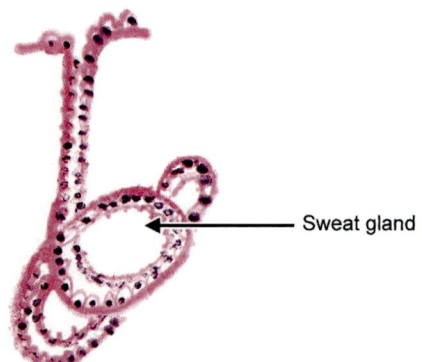

Fig. 4.2: Simple coiled tubular gland (20X)

Glands

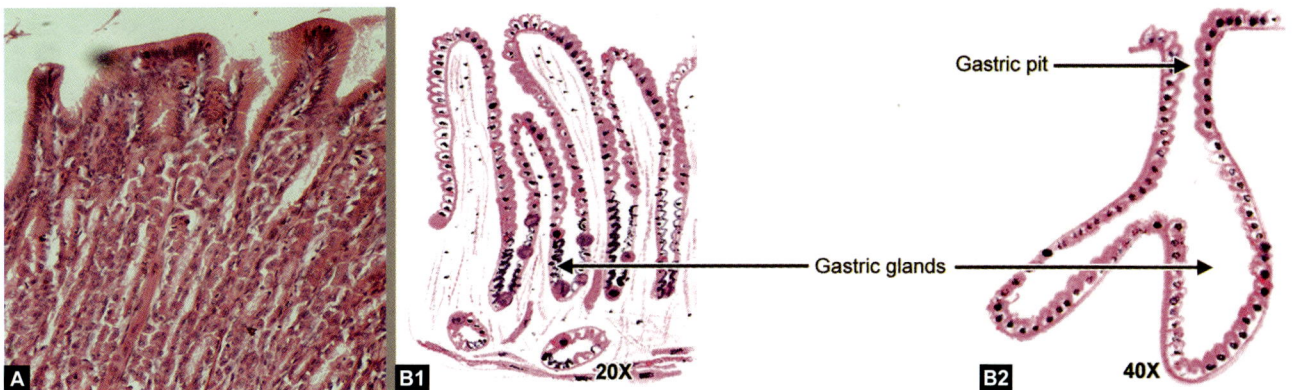

Figs 4.3A and B: (A) Microphotograph: Simple branched tubular gland; (B1, B2) Diagrammatic representation

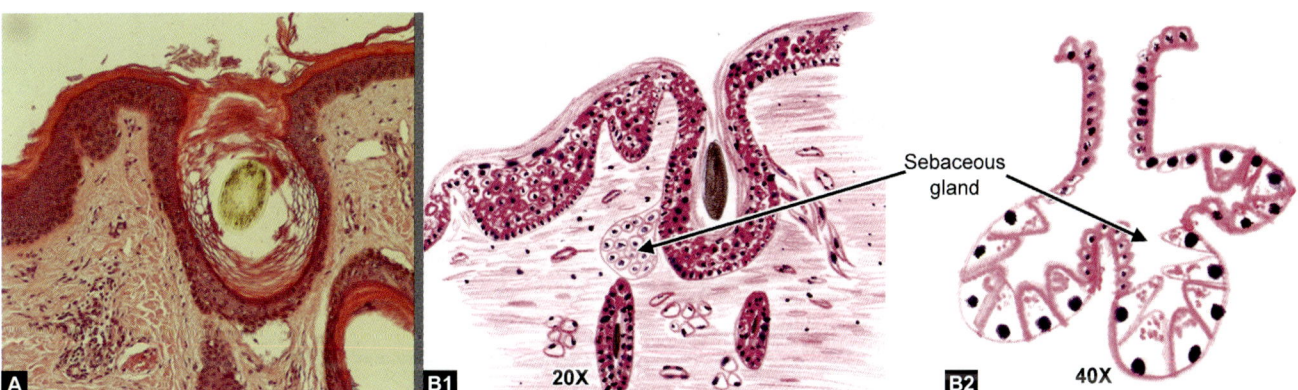

Figs 4.4A and B: (A) Microphotograph: Simple branched acinar gland; (B1, B2) Diagrammatic representation

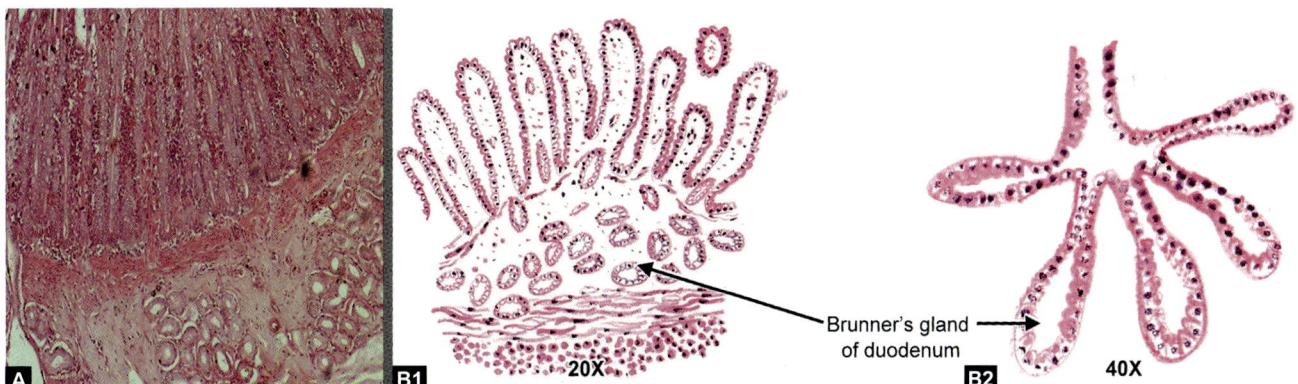

Figs 4.5A and B: (A) Microphotograph: Compound tubular gland; (B1, B2) Diagrammatic representation

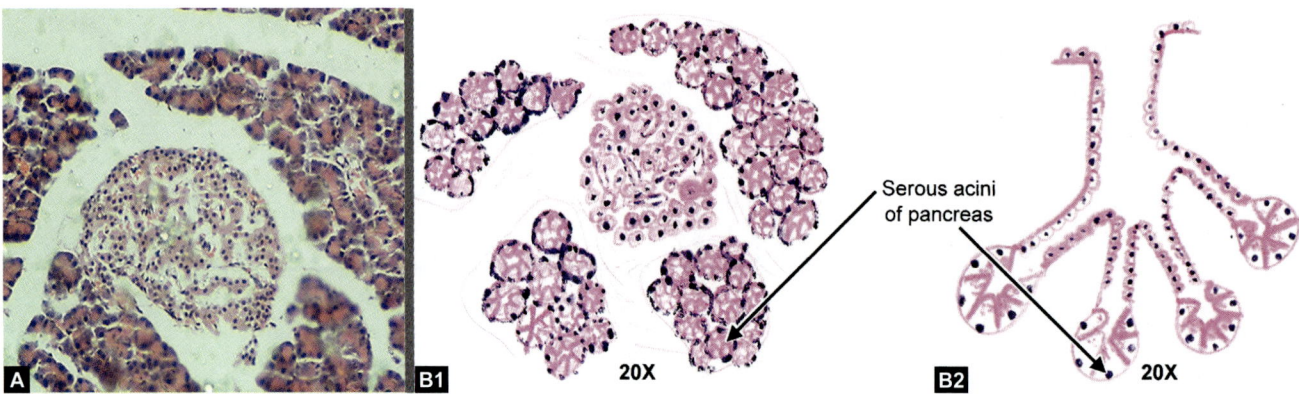

Figs 4.6A and B: (A) Microphotograph: Compound acinar gland; (B1, B2) Diagrammatic representation

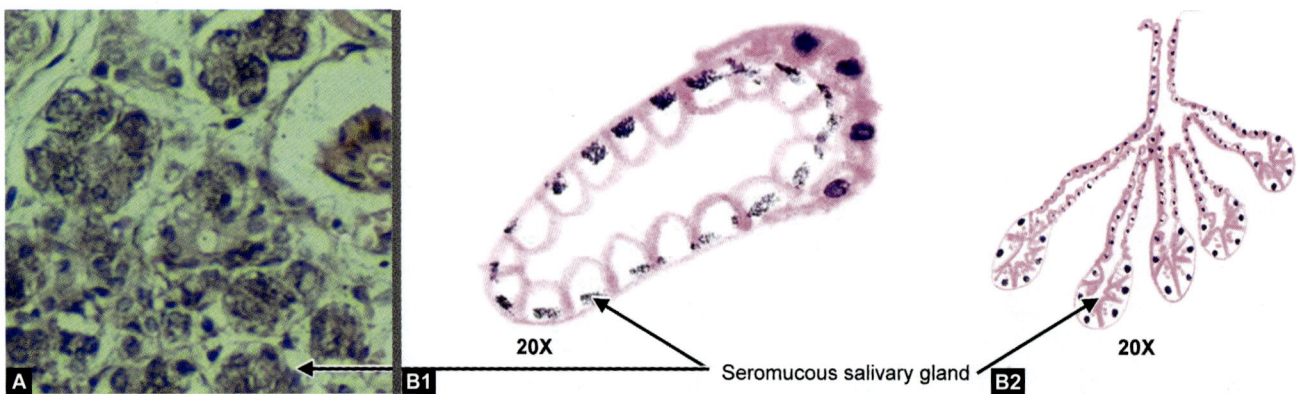

Figs 4.7A and B: (A) Microphotograph: Compound tubuloacinar gland; (B1, B2) Diagrammatic representation

CHAPTER 5

Connective Tissue

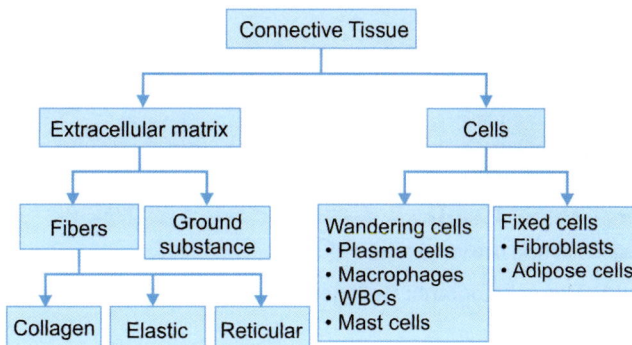

Tissue that fills the intercellular space between more specialized elements, supports and holds them together is called *Connective tissue*.

CELLS

Mesenchymal cells, fibroblasts, fibrocytes, adipose cells, reticular cells, pigment cells, macrophages, mast cells and plasma cells.

FIBERS

- *Collagen fibers:*
  - Most numerous
  - Run in bundles which do not branch
  - Acidophilic in staining
- *Elastic fibers:*
  - Less frequent than collagen
  - Fine and run singly
  - Branch and anastomose freely
- *Reticular fibers:*
  - Are of small length
  - Branching and anastomosing
  - Specially stained by silver stain.

TABLE 5.1: Classification of connective tissue

Embryonic connective tissue	Connective tissue proper	Specialized connective tissue

• Mesenchymal
• Mucous connective tissue
	• Loose connective tissue
	• Dense connective tissue
	  – Irregular
	  – Regular
		• Cartilage
		• Bone
		• Adipose tissue
		• Blood
		• Lymphatic tissue

12 Atlas of Histology for Medical Students

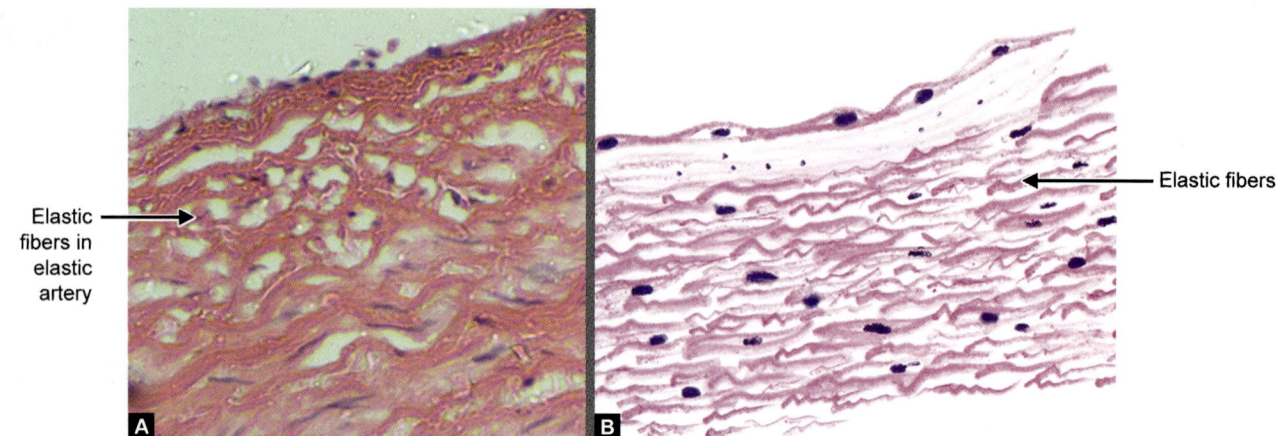

Figs 5.1A and B: (A) Microphotograph: Elastic fibers (40X); (B) Diagrammatic representation

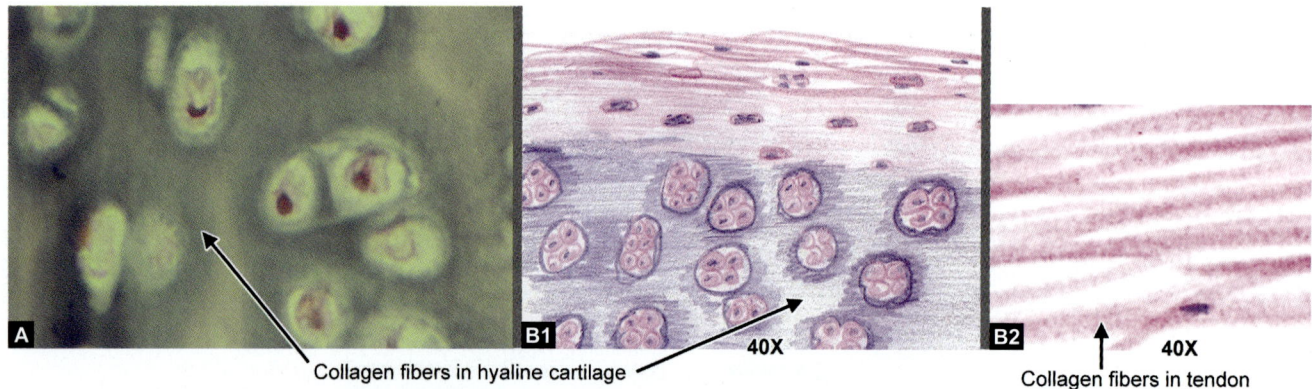

Figs 5.2A and B: (A) Microphotograph: Collagen fibers; (B1, B2) Diagrammatic representation

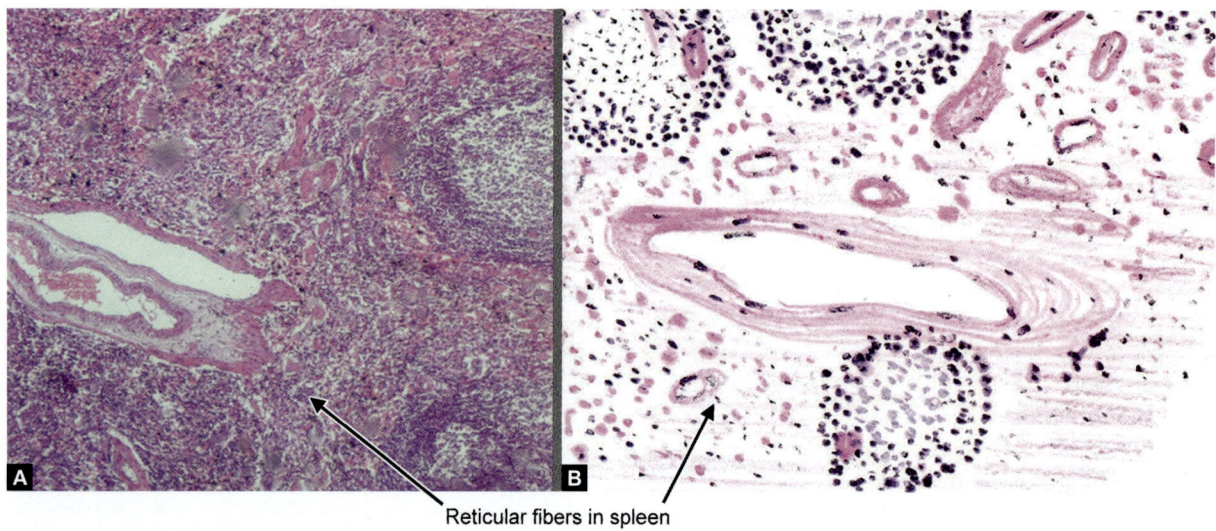

Figs 5.3A and B: (A) Microphotograph: Reticular fibers (40X); (B) Diagrammatic representation

Connective Tissue

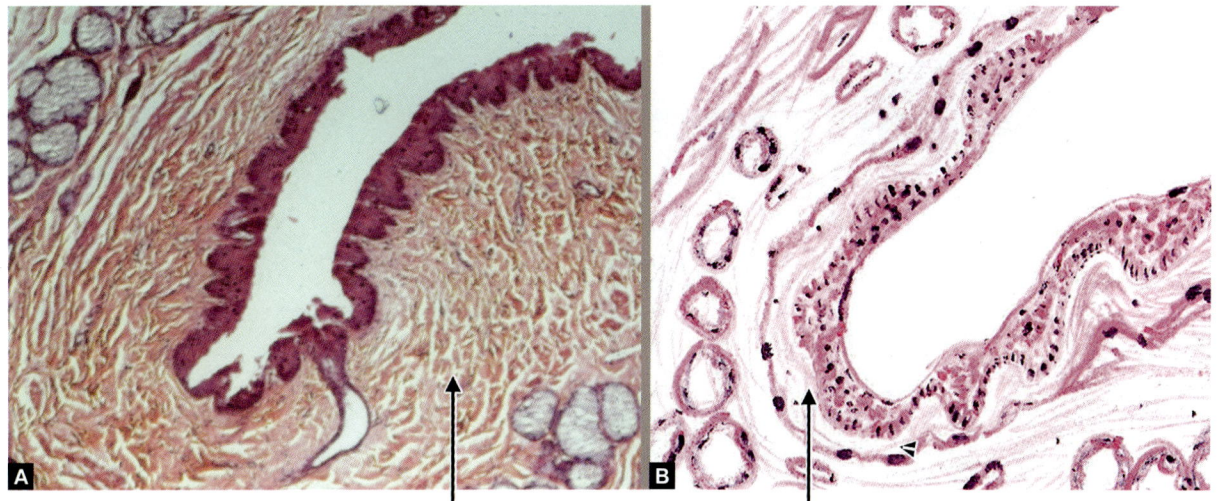

Figs 5.4A and B: (A) Microphotograph: Loose connective tissue (20X); (B) Diagrammatic representation

Lamina propria in esophagus (in all tissues deep to epithelium)

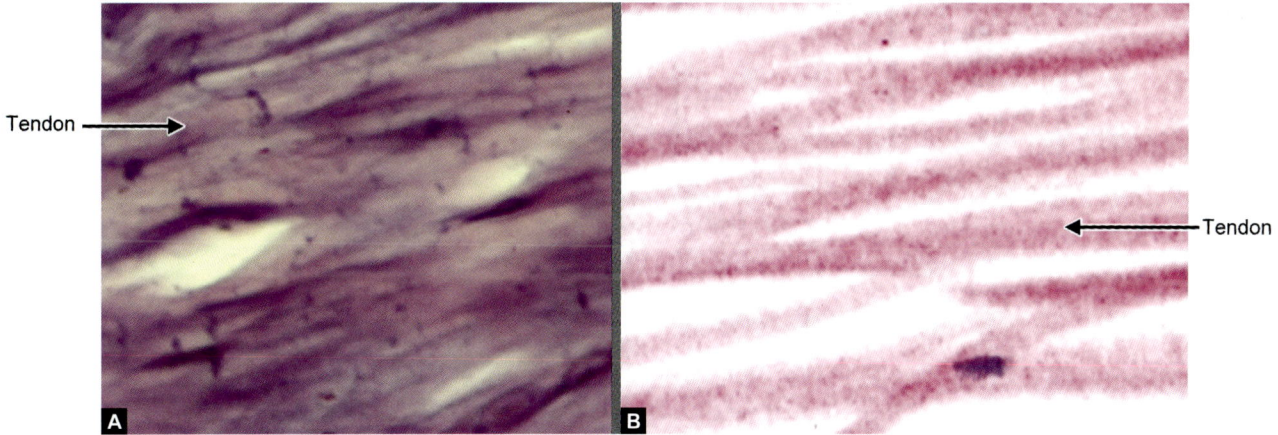

Figs 5.5A and B: (A) Microphotograph: Dense regular connective tissue (20X); (B) Diagrammatic representation

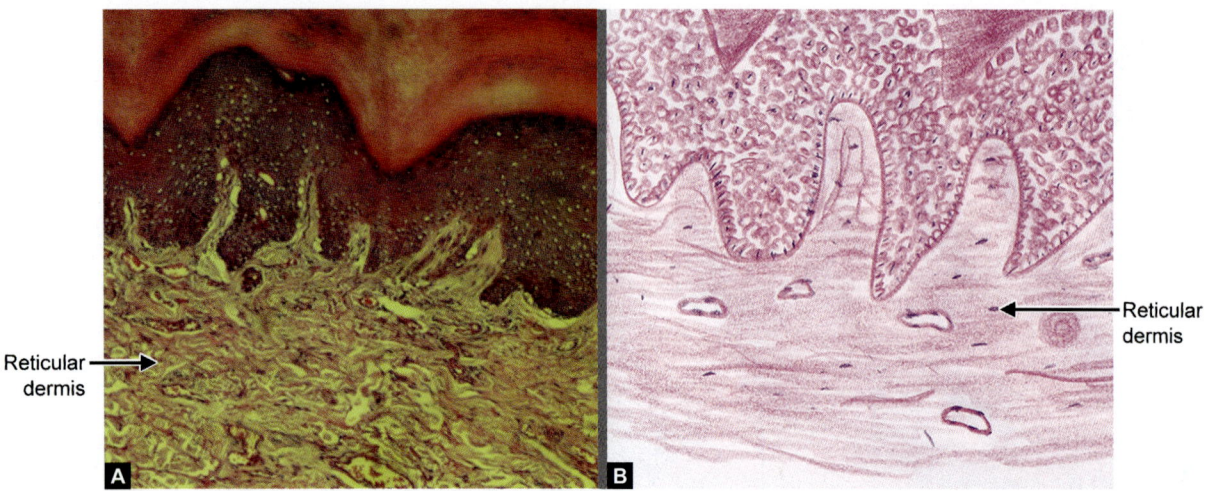

Figs 5.6A and B: (A) Microphotograph: Dense irregular connective tissue (20X); (B) Diagrammatic representation

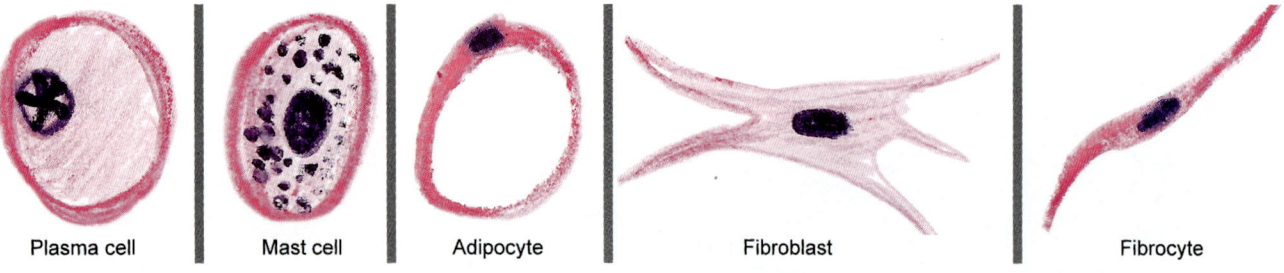

Fig. 5.7: Connective tissue cells (40X)

CHAPTER 6

Cartilage

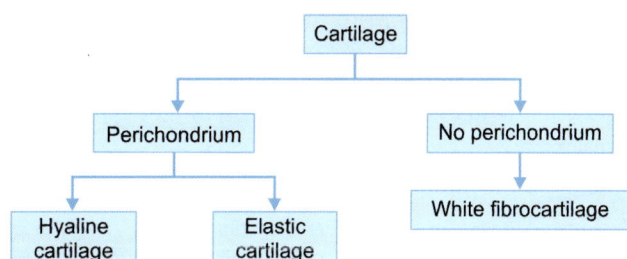

SPECIALIZED CONNECTIVE TISSUE

Hyaline Cartilage

- Perichondrium: Fibrous layer—collagen fibers, fibroblasts
  Cellular layer—Chondroblasts
- Isogenous group of chondrocytes in lacuna
- Homogenous basophilic matrix: Collagen fibers (Type II) not visible as refractive index same as ground substance (proteoglycans and structural glycosaminoglycans)
- For example: Costal cartilage, nose, larynx (thyroid, cricoid, arytenoids), trachea, articular cartilage (does not have perichondrium)
- Can undergo calcification.

Elastic Cartilage

- Perichondrium: Fibrous layer—Collagen fibers, fibroblasts
  Cellular layer—Chondroblasts
- Single chondrocyte in lacuna
- Matrix: Numerous elastic fibers
- For example: External ear, auditory tube, epiglottis, larynx
- Resistant to calcification
- **Should be differentiated from tendon (chondrocytes in fibrocartilage are rounded, present in lacunae, while in tendon the fibroblasts/cytes are flattened and elongated).**

White Fibrocartilage

- Perichondrium: Absent
- Matrix: Dense collagen fibers in parallel arrangement
- Rows of single chondrocytes in lacunae
- For example: Intervertebral disc, Symphysis pubis.

16 Atlas of Histology for Medical Students

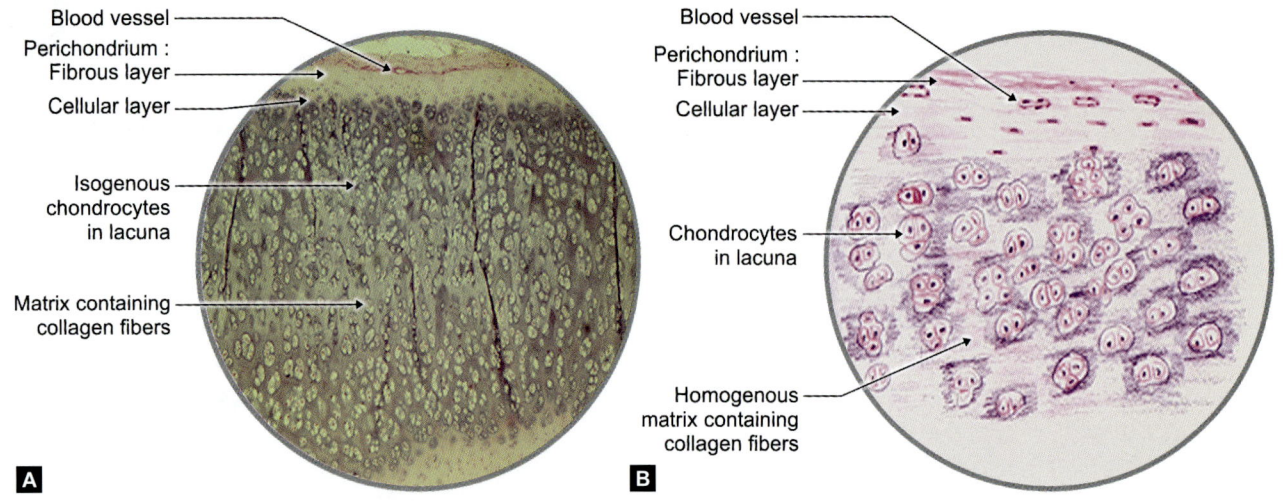

Figs 6.1A and B: (A) Microphotograph: Hyaline cartilage (4X); (B) Diagrammatic representation

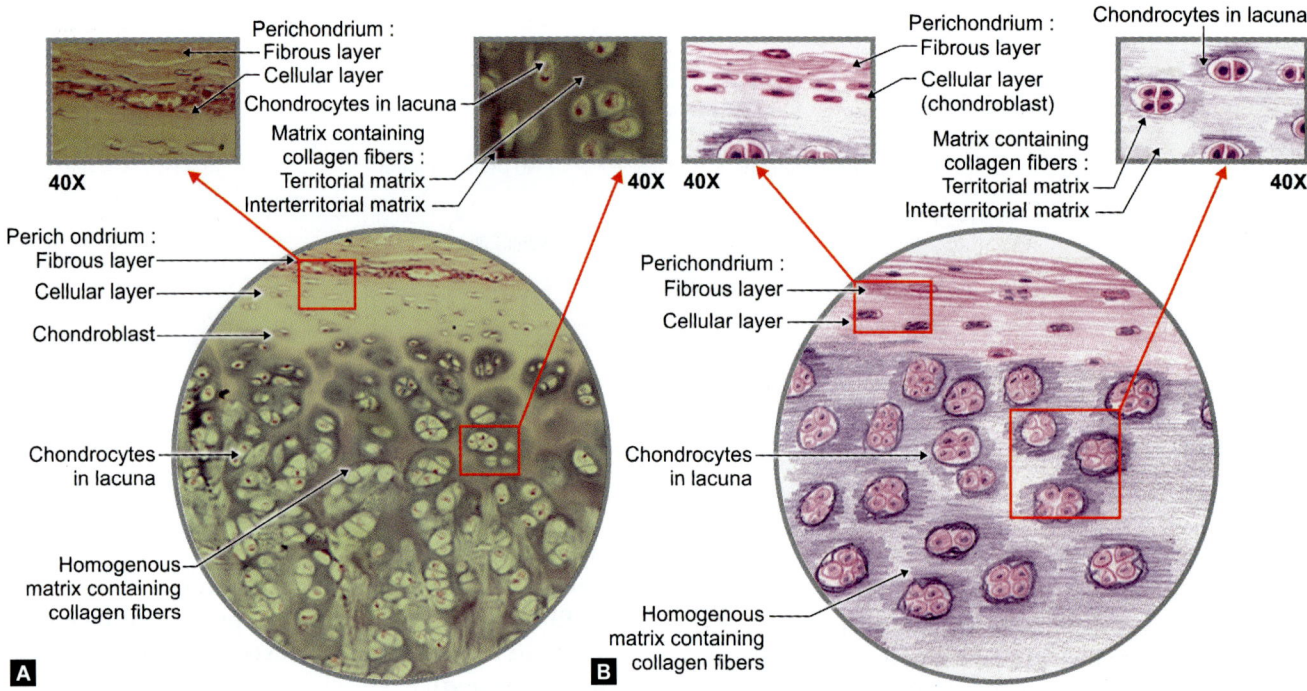

Figs 6.2A and B: (A) Microphotograph: Hyaline cartilage (20X); (B) Diagrammatic representation

Cartilage 17

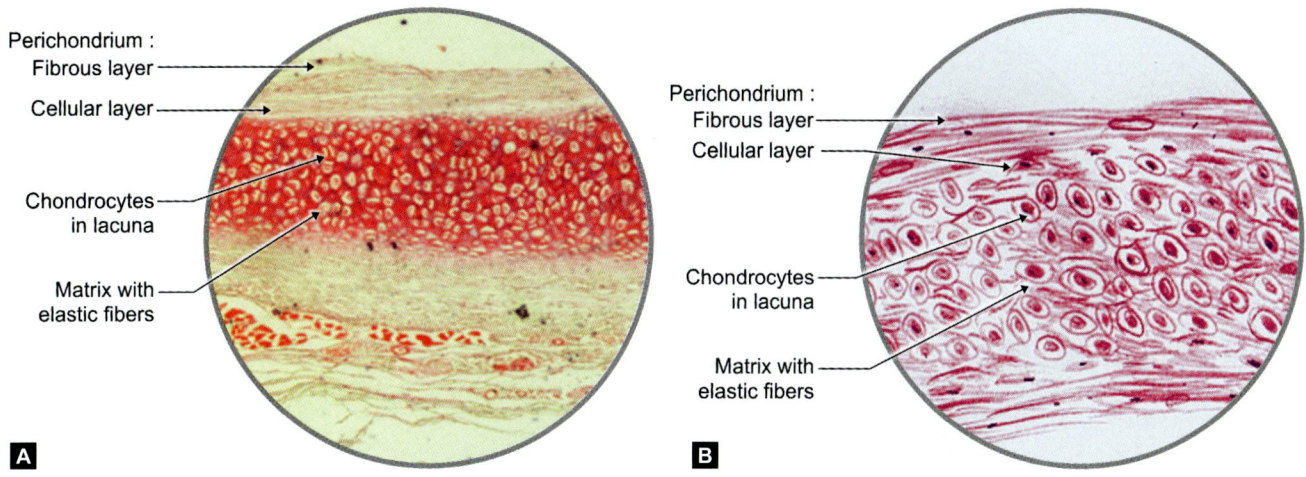

Figs 6.3A and B: (A) Microphotograph: Elastic cartilage (4X); (B) Diagrammatic representation

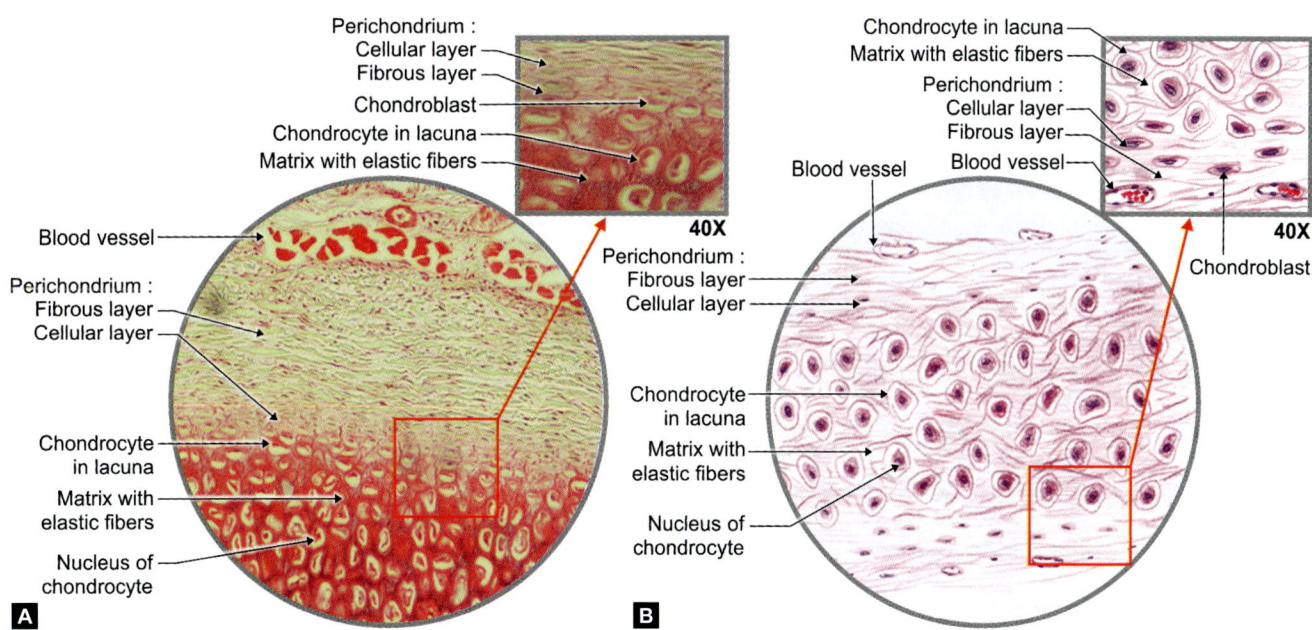

Figs 6.4A and B: (A) Microphotograph: Elastic cartilage (20X); (B) Diagrammatic representation

18 Atlas of Histology for Medical Students

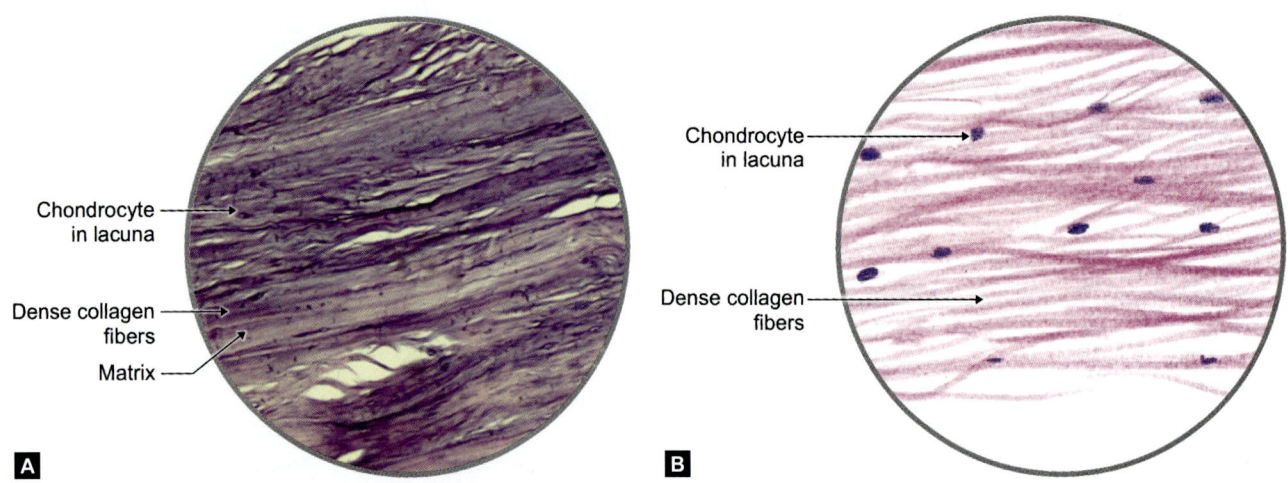

Figs 6.5A and B: (A) Microphotograph: White fibrocartilage (4X); (B) Diagrammatic representation

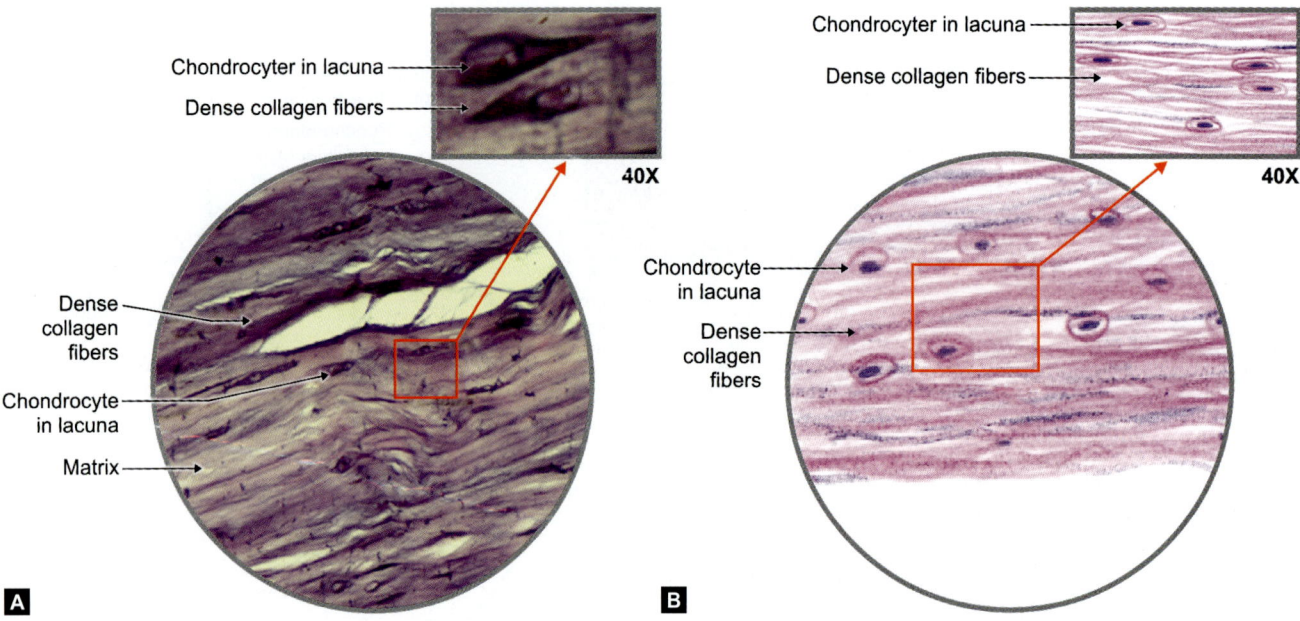

Figs 6.6A and B: (A) Microphotograph: White fibrocartilage (20X); (B) Diagrammatic representation

CHAPTER 7

Bone

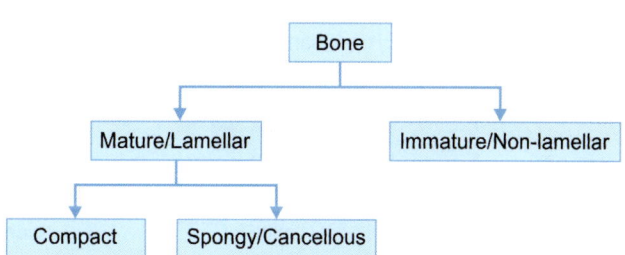

- One of the four basic tissues of the body
- Highly specialized living cells with extracellular matrix
- Mineralization of matrix (calcium phosphate- hydroxyapatite crystals- $[Ca_{10}(PO_4)_6(OH)_2]$
- For support, protection, homeostatic regulation of blood calcium levels
- Outer surfaces of bone covered by periosteum (outer dense connective tissue sheath with inner cellular osteoprogenitor cells layer)
- Blood supply to bone tissue is centrifugal.

COMPACT

- Cylindrical unit: Called osteons (Haversian system)
- Osteons: Lamellae in radial pattern surrounding a central canal
- Lamellae: Concentric, interstitial, circumferential lamellae
- Volkmann's canals are channels connecting haversian canals
- High proportion of bone matrix as compared to spongy bone.

SPONGY

- Similar in structure to compact bone
- Tissue arranged as trabeculae or spicules with spaces filled with bone marrow
- More soft tissue/marrow spaces that are interconnecting as compared to matrix
- Matrix is lamellated.

ENDOCHONDRAL OSSIFICATION

The process of bone formation is ossification. In endochondral ossification a cartilage model is replaced by bone. The epiphyseal plate of long bone is the best example of growing bone. The slide of developing bone shows following zones.

1. *Zone of resting cartilage:* Chondrocytes are small and flat. This is a reserve zone of normal hyaline cartilage in

which chondrocytes are distributed in lacunae singly or in groups.
2. *Zone of proliferation:* This is a zone of cartilage growth. Cells are larger and show mitotic activity. They multiply and arrange in parallel columns separated by bars of matrix.
3. *Zone of maturation:* Cells increase in size and secrete alkaline phosphatase. Chondrocytes hypertrophy by swelling of nucleus and cytoplasm and lacunae enlarge.
4. *Zone of calcification:* Calcium salts are deposited in the matrix of the cartilage. Chondrocytes die leaving lacunae or empty spaces, with dead and dying cells. This is chondrolysis.
5. *Zone of ossification:* Blood vessels from the periosteum grow inside and the calcified matrix is replaced by bone matrix. Chondrogenic layer of periosteum is stimulated to differentiate into osteogenic layer from which osteoblast are formed

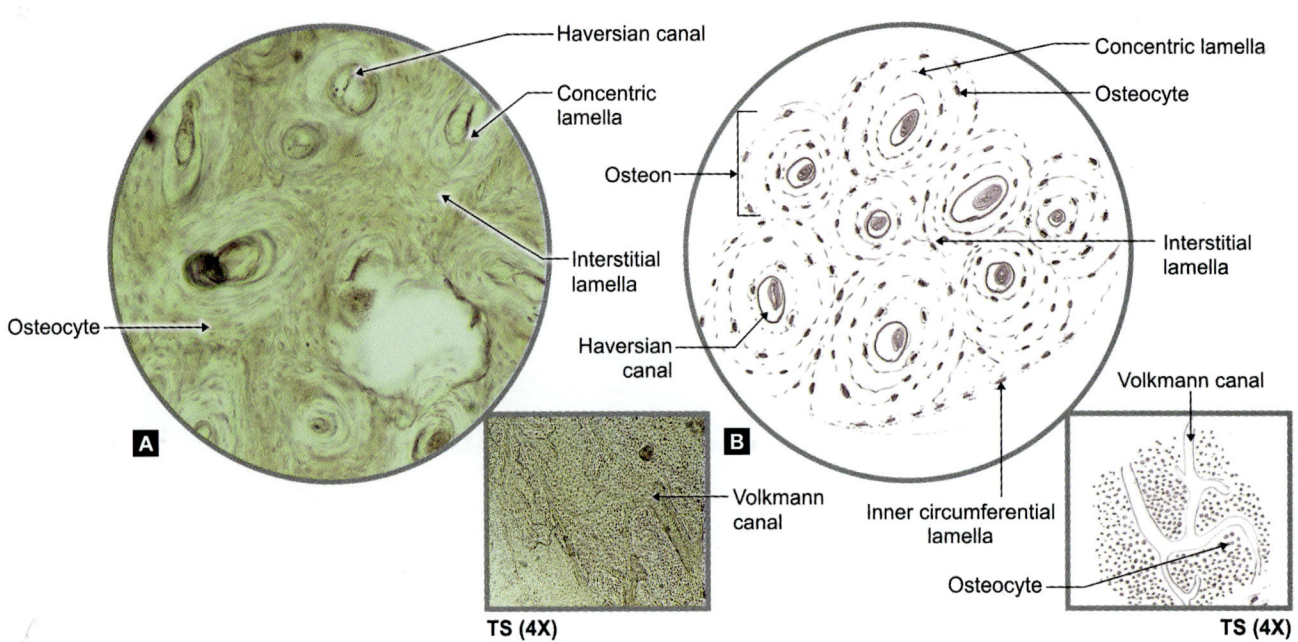

Figs 7.1A and B: (A) Microphotograph: Compact bone (4X); (B) Diagrammatic representation

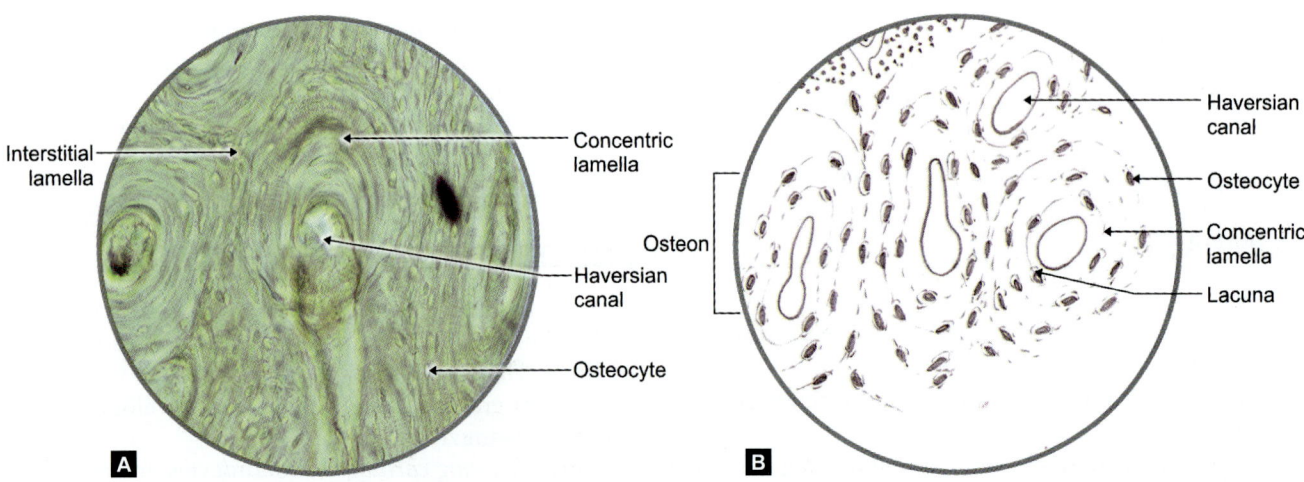

Figs 7.2A and B: (A) Microphotograph: Compact bone (20X); (B) Diagrammatic representation

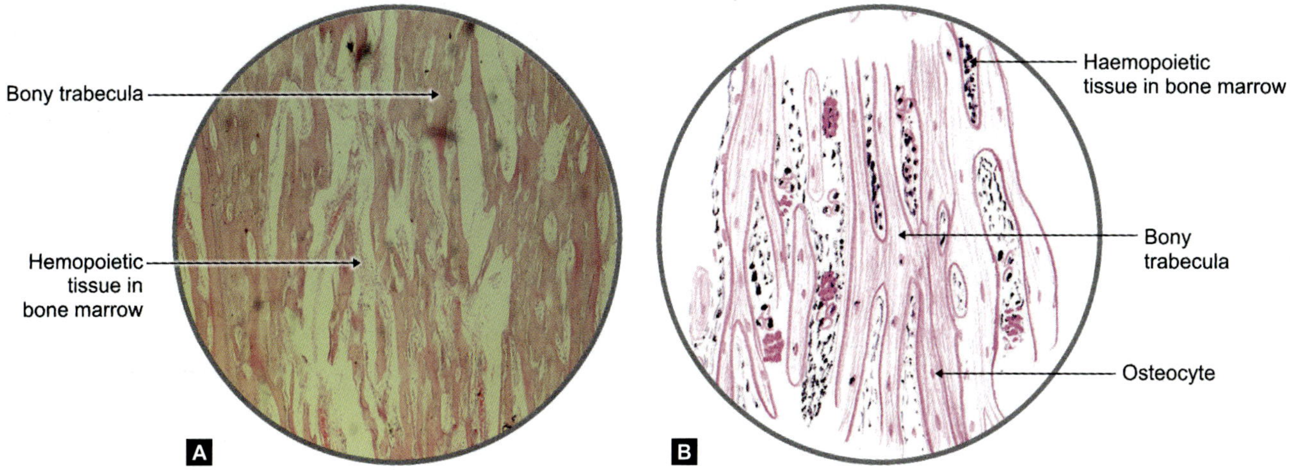

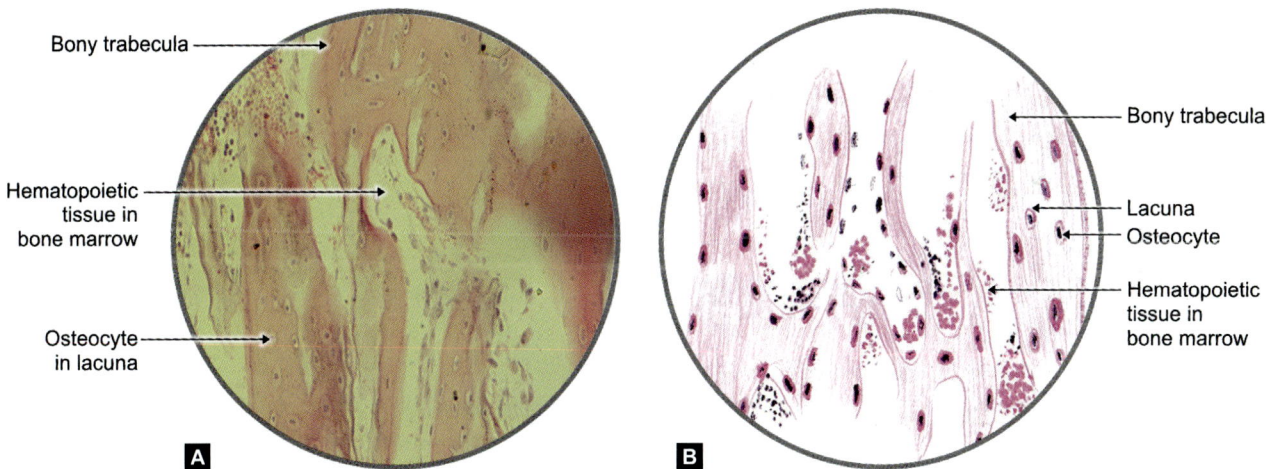

Figs 7.3A and B: (A) Microphotograph: Spongy bone (4X); (B) Diagrammatic representation

Figs 7.4A and B: (A) Microphotograph: Spongy bone (20X); (B) Diagrammatic representation

CHAPTER 8

Muscle

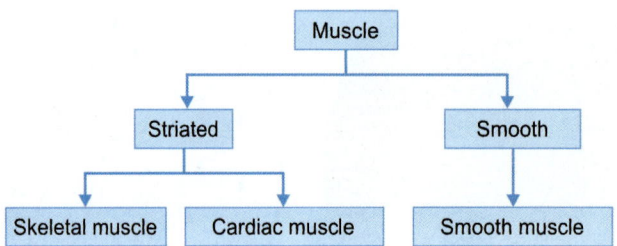

CONTRACTILE TISSUE

- One of the four basic tissues of the body
- Highly specialized cells with property to shorten/contract
- Covered by connective tissue (without inwards—Epimysium, perimysium, endomysium).

1. *Skeletal/voluntary*
   - Essentially word 'striated' refers to skeletal muscle
   - Related to skeleton
   - Generally voluntary in nature
   - Fibers are long and parallel without branching
   - Multinucleated (syncytium)
   - Dark and light transverse striations
   - Nuclei peripherally placed.

2. *Cardiac muscle*
   - Cells are joined together end to end by cell junctions forming the intercalated disks
   - Transverse striations
   - Fibers branch and anastomose
   - Involuntary in nature
   - Single centrally placed nucleus surrounded by perinuclear halo

3. *Smooth muscle*
   - Does not exhibit striations
   - Involuntary in nature (Contraction under control of autonomic nervous system)
   - Found in walls of hollow viscera, bood vessels etc,
   - Fibers have elongated tapering form (spindle shaped)
   - Single oval centrally placed nucleus.

Muscle 23

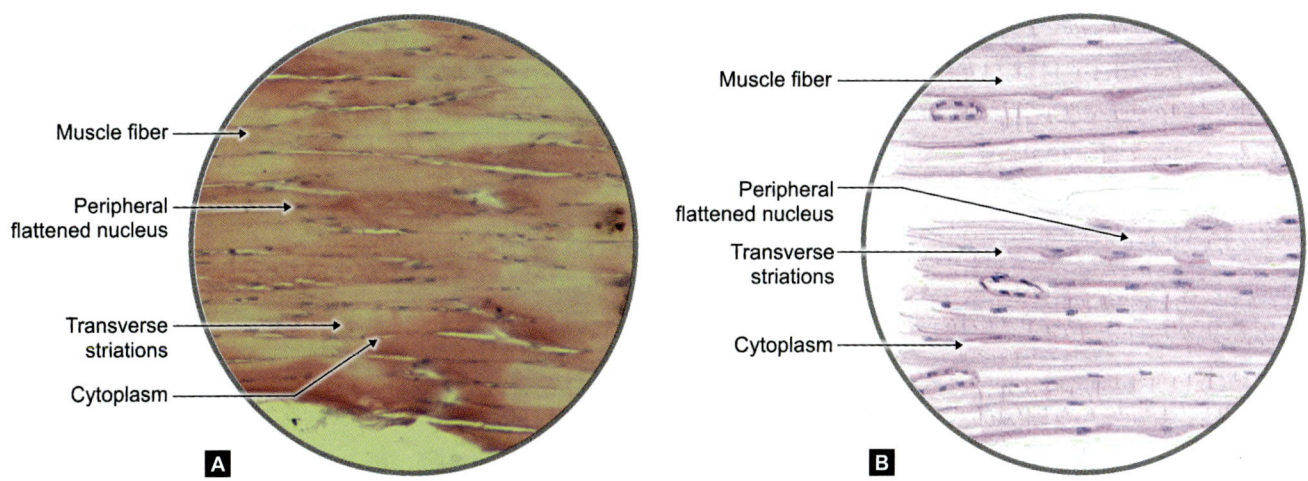

Figs 8.1A and B: (A) Microphotograph: Skeletal muscle (LS)(4X); (B) Diagrammatic representation

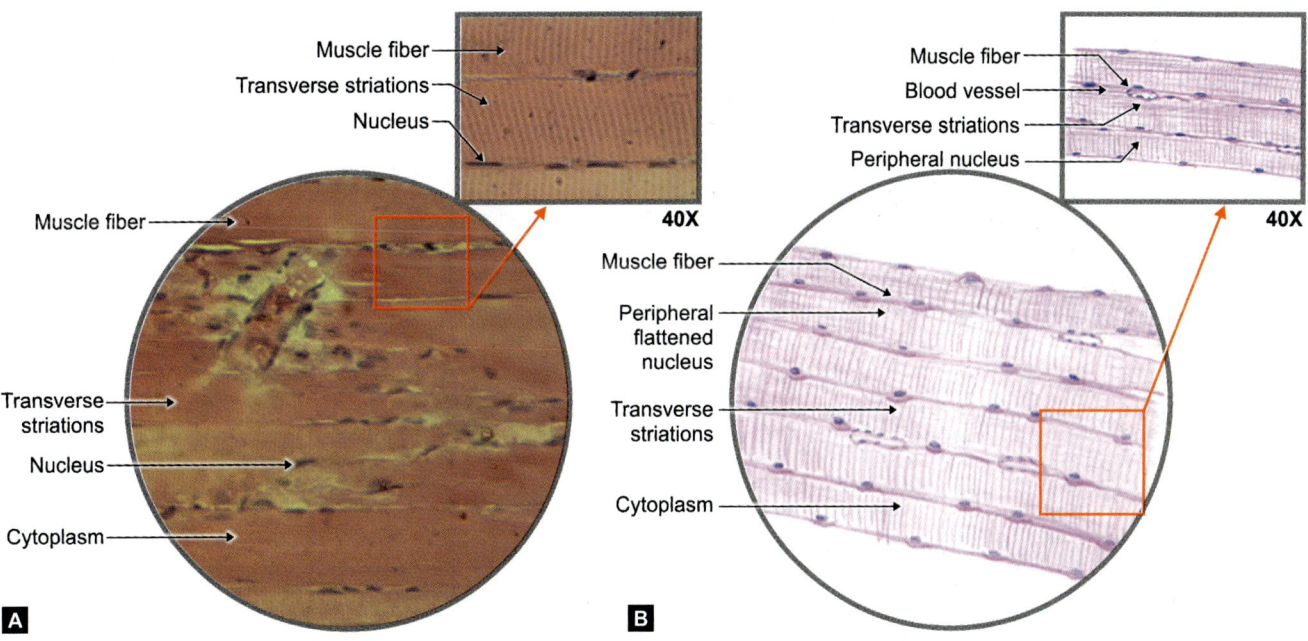

Figs 8.2A and B: (A) Microphotograph: Skeletal muscle (LS)(20X); (B) Diagrammatic representation

24 Atlas of Histology for Medical Students

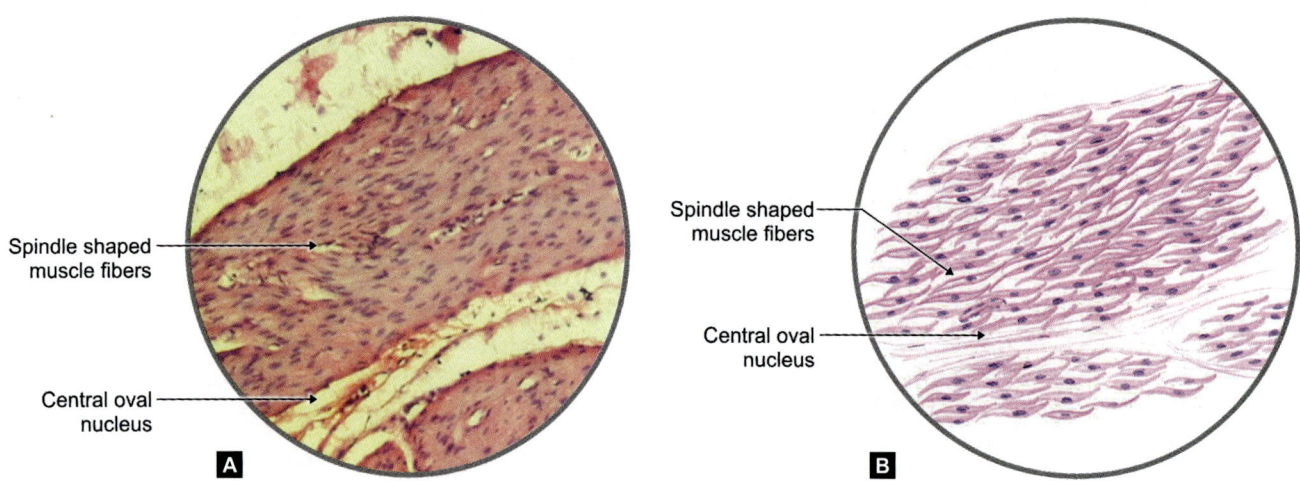

Figs 8.3A and B: (A) Microphotograph: Smooth muscle (LS)(4X); (B) Diagrammatic representation

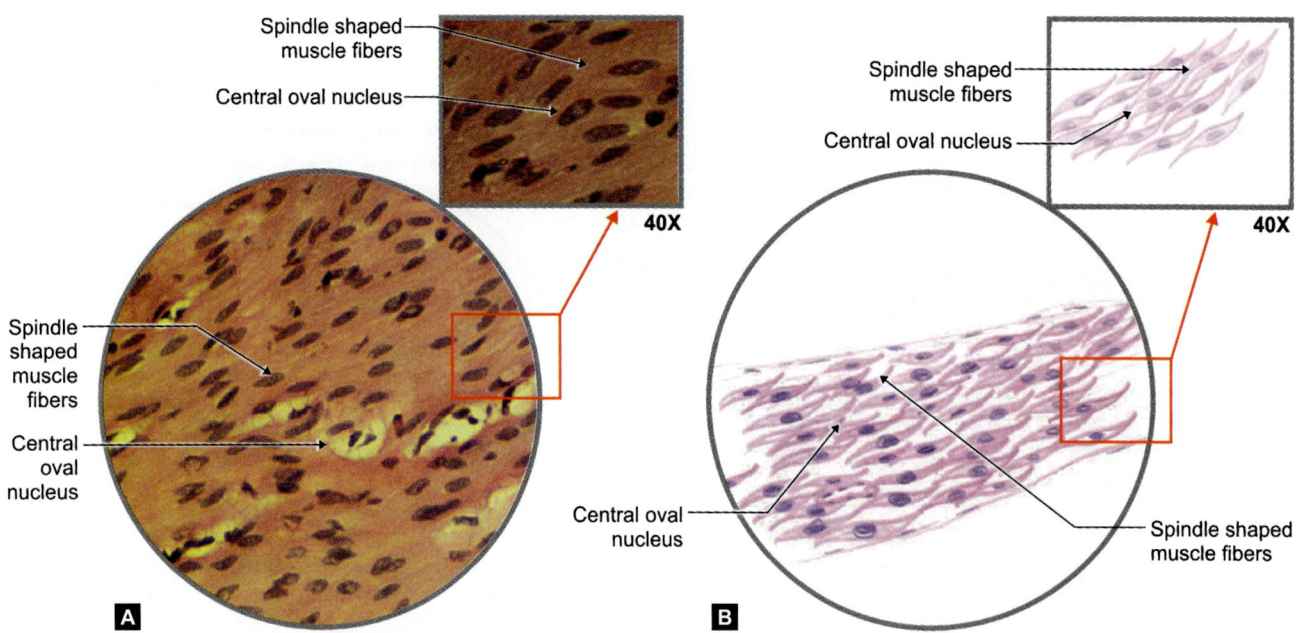

Figs 8.4A and B: (A) Microphotograph: Smooth muscle (LS)(20X); (B) Diagrammatic representation

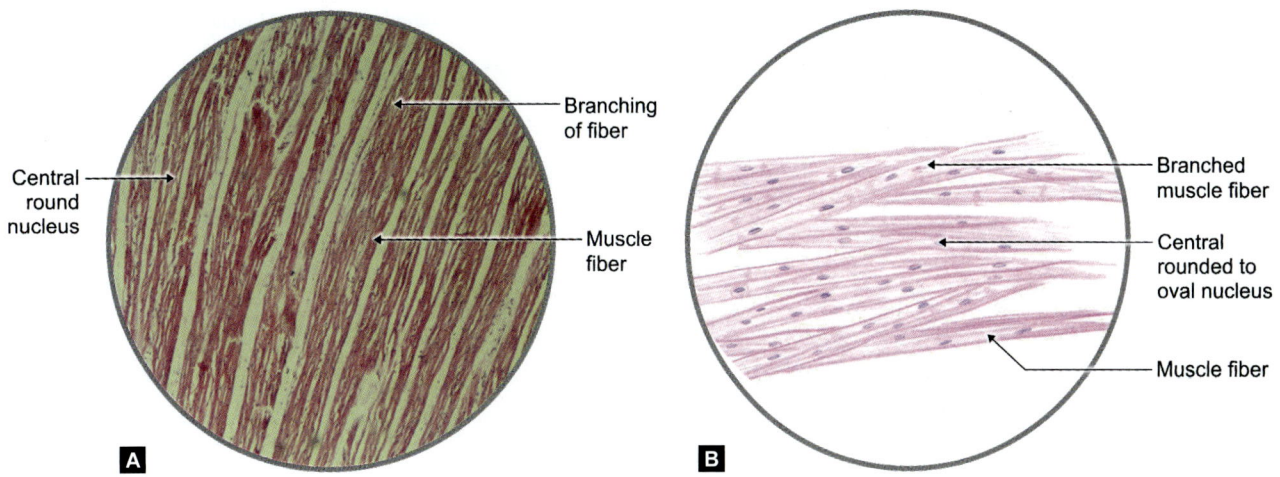

Figs 8.5A and B: (A) Microphotograph: Cardiac muscle (LS)(4X); (B) Diagrammatic representation

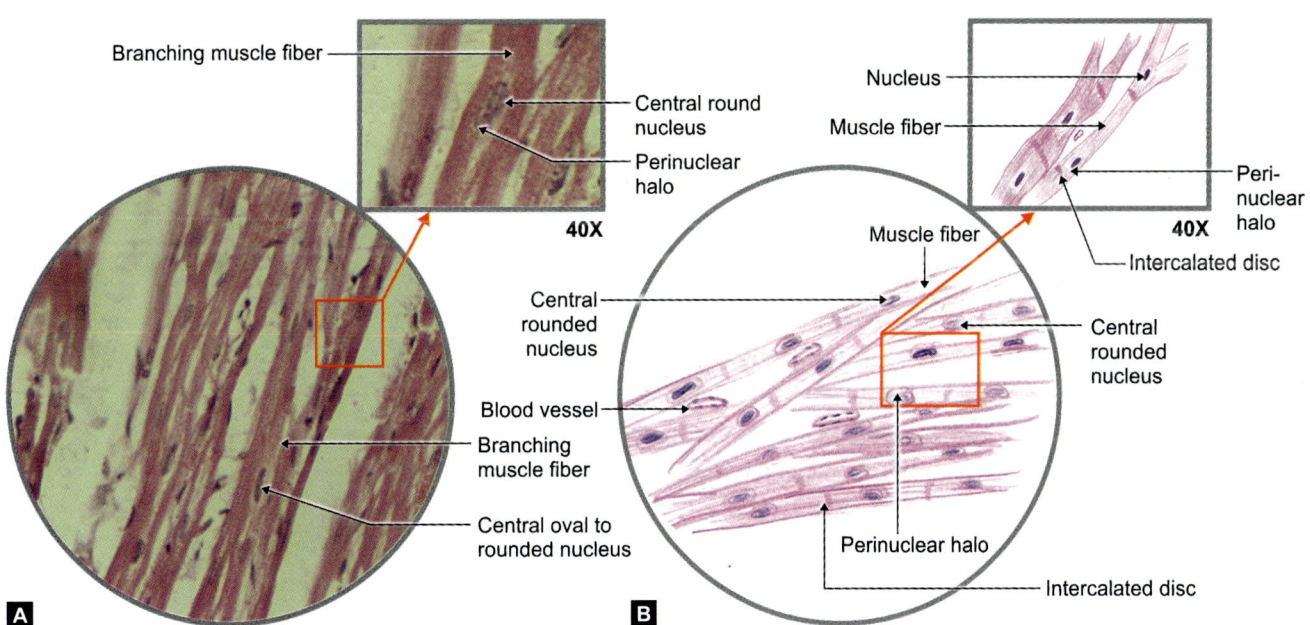

Figs 8.6A and B: (A) Microphotograph: Cardiac muscle (LS)(20X); (B) Diagrammatic representation

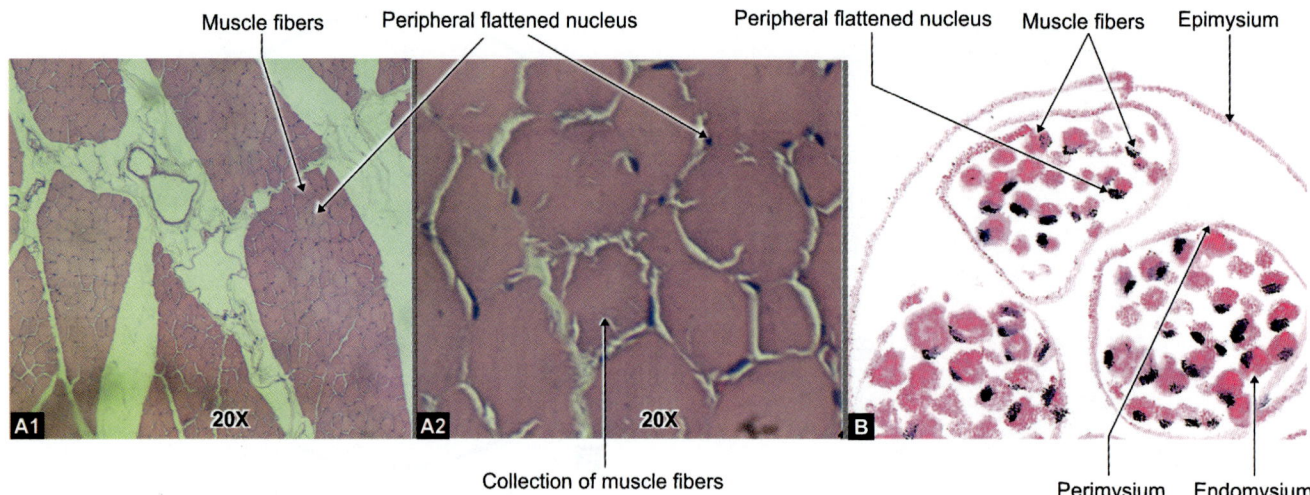

Figs 8.7A and B: (A1, A2) Microphotographs: Striated muscle (TS)(4X); (B) Diagrammatic representation

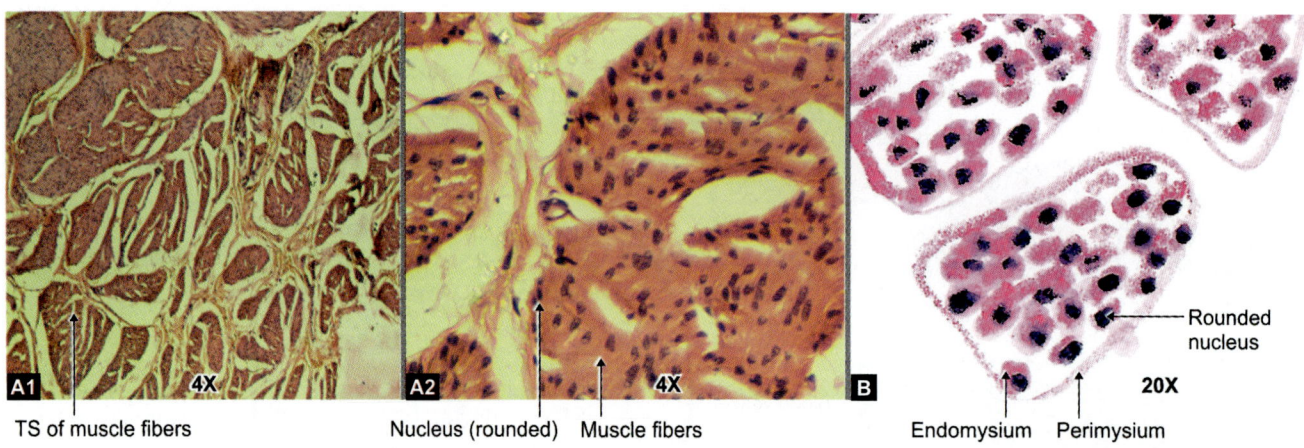

Figs 8.8A and B: (A1, A2) Microphotographs: Smooth muscle (TS)(4X); (B) Diagrammatic representation

CHAPTER 9

Nervous Tissue

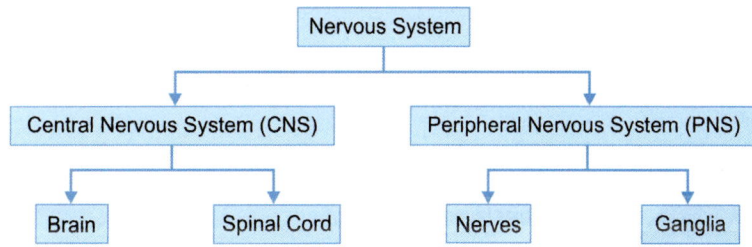

Nervous tissue consists of two types of cells:
  I. Neurons
  II. Supporting cells—
    In CNS- Neuroglia- Oligodendrocytes, Astrocytes, Microglia, ependymal cells
    In PNS—Schwann cells

Functionally nervous system consists of:
  I. Somatic
  II. Autonomic

Anatomically the nervous system consists of:
  I. Central nervous system (CNS): Consists of brain and spinal cord
  II. Peripheral nervous system (PNS): Consists of cranial, spinal and peripheral nerves, and ganglia.

CENTRAL NERVOUS TISSUE

Cerebrum

- Consists of cortex (covered by pia mater) which contains gray matter
- White matter is present on the inner aspect
- Six layers of cortex consists of (from outer to inner):

1. *Plexiform (Molecular layer):* Consists of fibers, few horizontal cells of cajal and neuroglial cells.
2. *Outer granular layer (Small pyramidal):* Consists of small pyramidal cells, granule or stellate cells.
3. *Outer pyramidal layer (Medium pyramidal):* Cells medium in size with typical pyramidal shape.
4. *Inner granular layer:* Many granule cells.
5. *Inner pyramidal layer:* Pyramidal shaped cells **(motor area contains Giant pyramidal cells called—Betz cells).**
6. Layer of polymorphic cells of different shape.

Cerebellum

- Consists of cortex (covered by pia mater) which contains gray matter
- White matter is present on the inner aspect
- Cerebellum has arbor vitae appearance
- Cerebellar cortex consists of 3 layers:
  - *Molecular layer (Outermost):* Basket cells
  - *Purkinje cell layer:* Flask shaped cell bodies of Purkinje cells
  - *Granular layer:* Showing small nuclei of granule cells
- White matter contains nerve fibers.

Spinal Cord

- Transverse section of spinal cord shows gray matter inside (butterfly shaped—containing neuronal cell bodies) and white matter containing nerve fibers forming tracts
- Butterfly shaped gray matter has dorsal (sensory) and ventral (motor) horns
- Ventral horn contains large cell bodies of multipolar neurons with prominent nucleolus.

Peripheral

Nerve Trunk

- Composed of bundle of nerve fibers
- Covered with connective tissue (within outwards—Endoneurium, Perineurium, Epineurium)
- Transverse section (TS) consists of cross section of myelinated nerve fibers containing centrally placed axon with surrounding myelin space
- Longitudinal section (LS) consists of bundles of nerve fibers in which there is a centrally placed axon with surrounding myelin space and nodes of Ranvier appearing as constrictions in neurilemma.

Dorsal Root Ganglion

- Pseudounipolar neurons with bundles of nerve fibers in between them
- Bodies of nerve cells extremely rounded
- Central nucleus is large pale staining (vesicular)
- Single prominent nucleolus
- Each rounded cell body lined by a single layer of flattened capsular cells/satellite cells.

Sympathetic Ganglion

- Similar to spinal ganglia with respect to connective tissue framework
- Multipolar neurons so irregular and less distinct contour
- Less uniform layer of capsule cells
- Smaller than those of spinal ganglia
- Eccentrically placed nucleus with prominent central nucleolus.

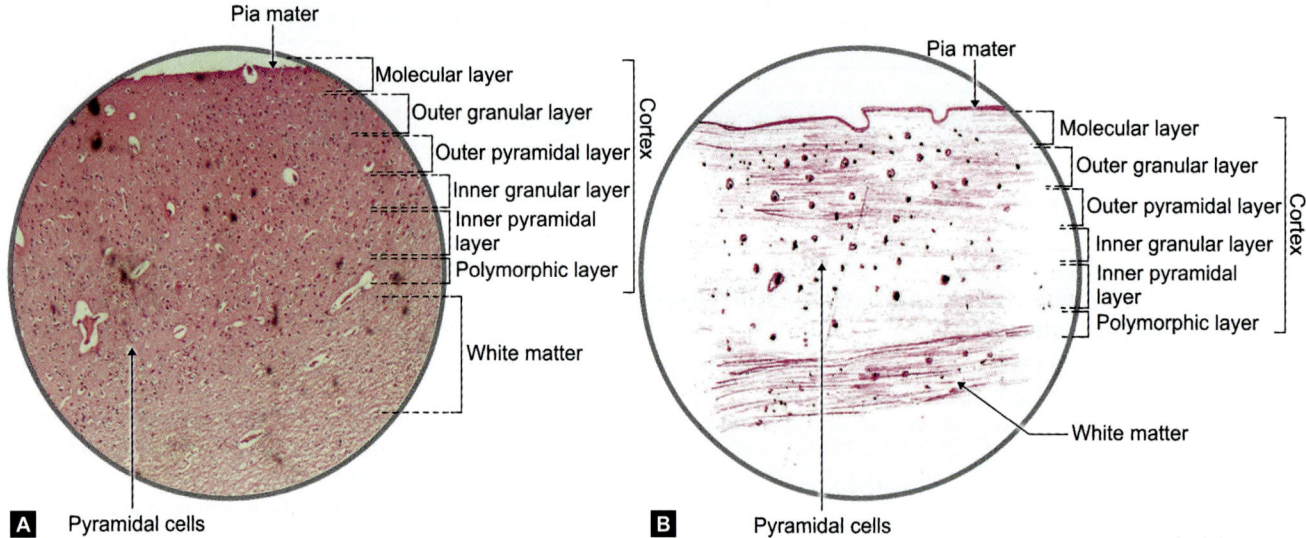

Figs 9.1A and B: (A) Microphotograph: Cerebrum (4X); (B) Diagrammatic representation

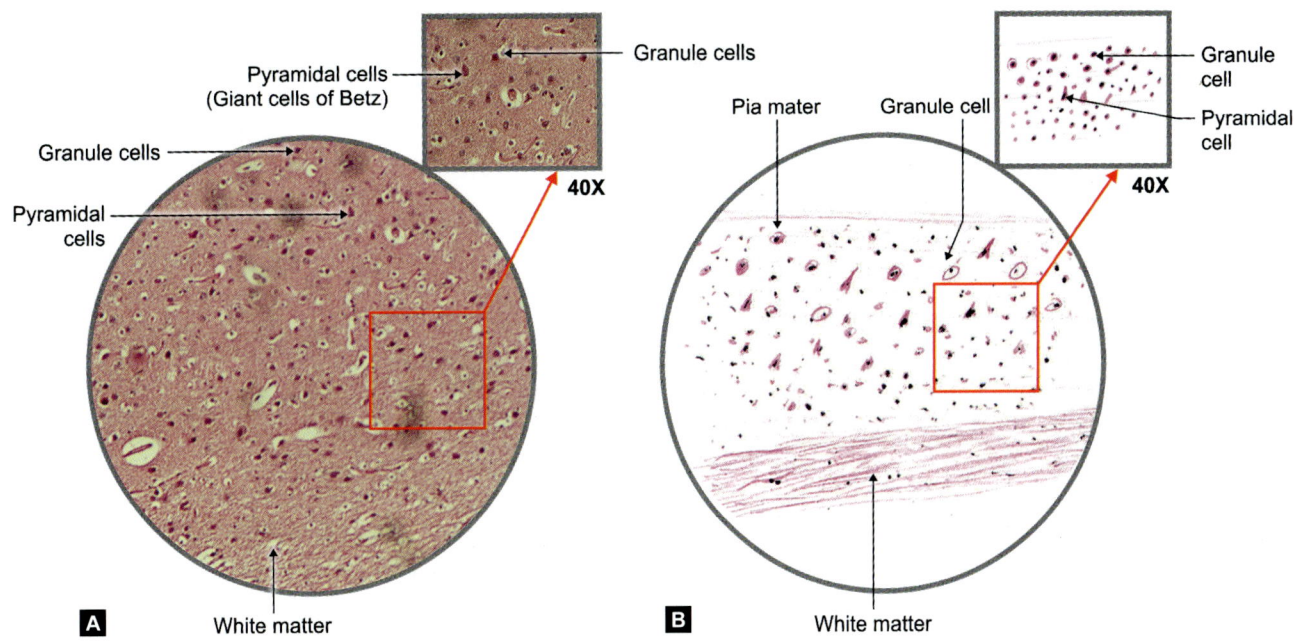

Figs 9.2A and B: (A) Microphotograph: Cerebrum (20X); (B) Diagrammatic representation

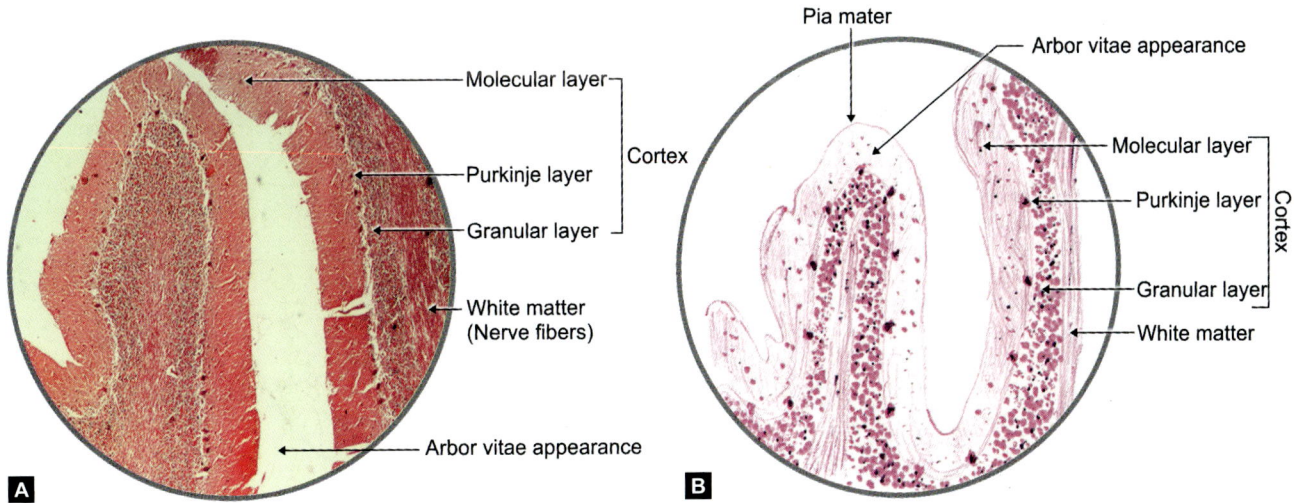

Figs 9.3A and B: (A) Microphotograph: Cerebellum (4X); (B) Diagrammatic representation

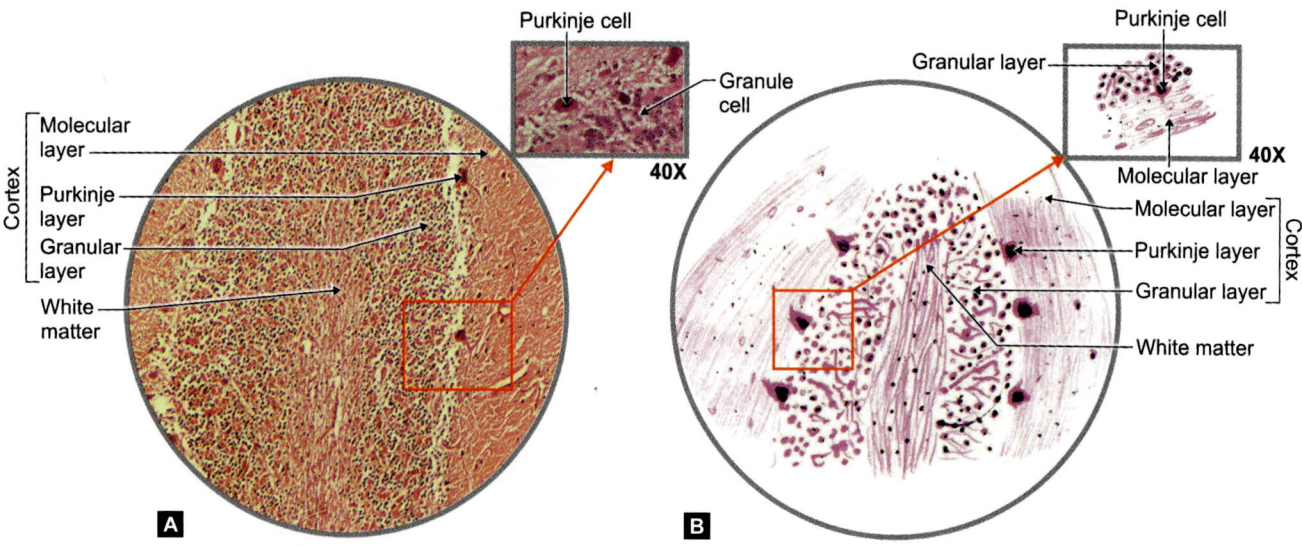

Figs 9.4A and B: (A) Microphotograph: Cerebellum (20X); (B) Diagrammatic representation

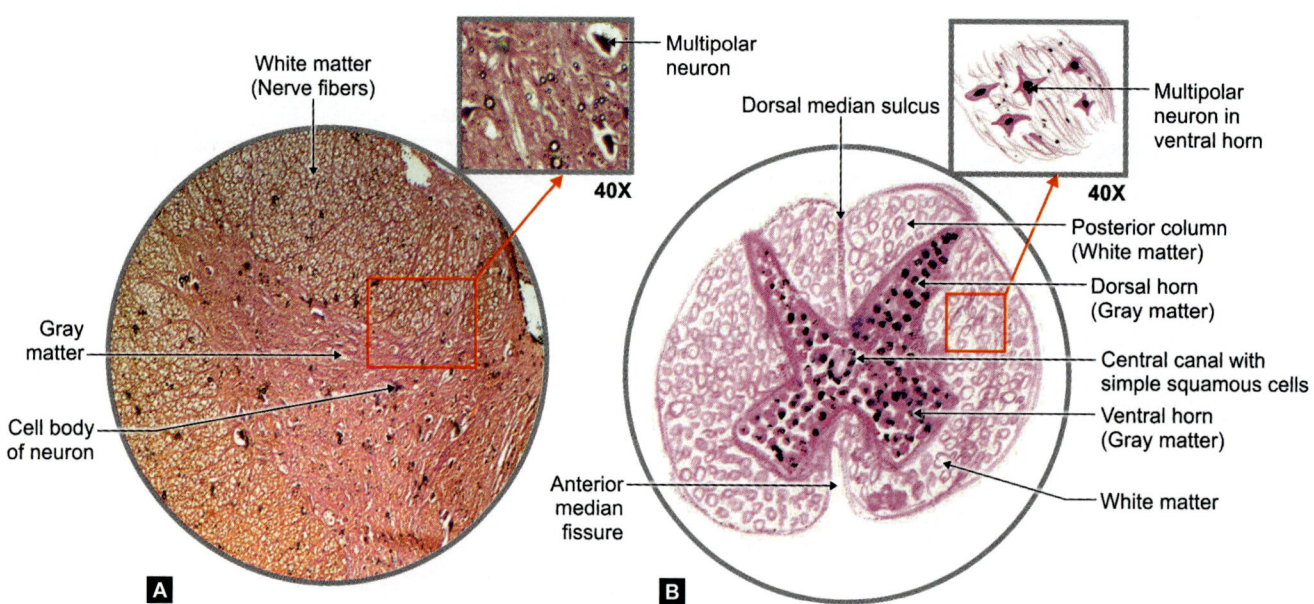

Figs 9.5A and B: (A) Microphotograph: Spinal cord (4X); (B) Diagrammatic representation

Nervous Tissue

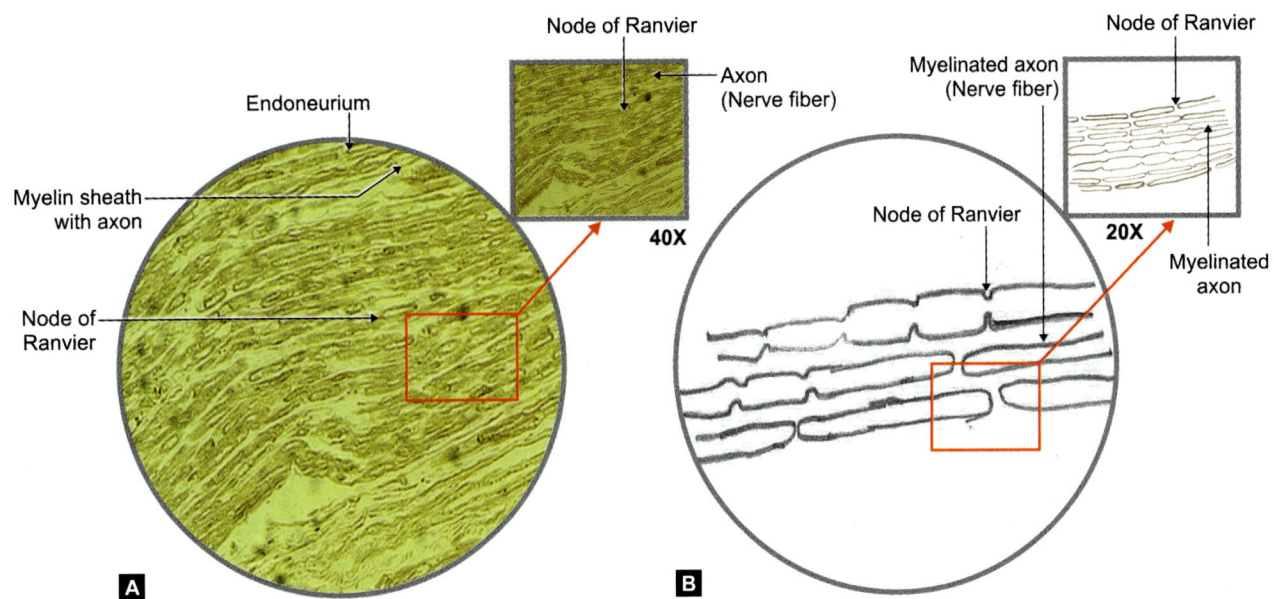

Figs 9.6A and B: (A) Microphotograph: Nerve trunk LS (4X); (B) Diagrammatic representation

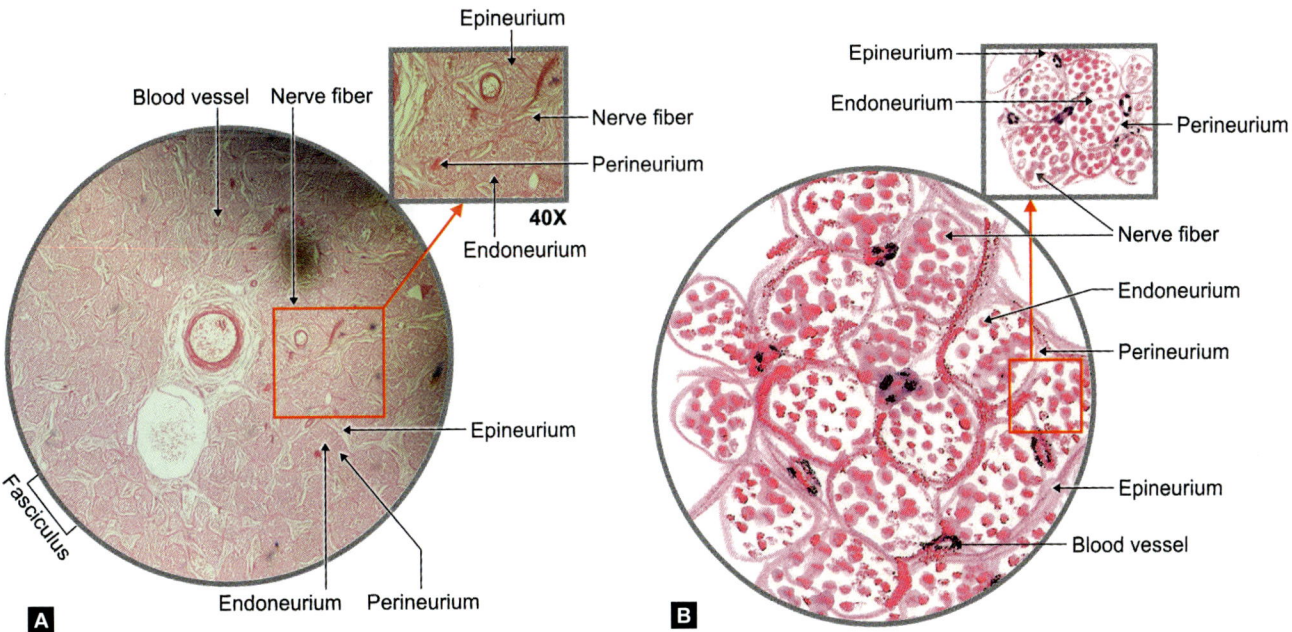

Figs 9.7A and B: (A) Microphotograph: Nerve trunk TS (4X); (B) Diagrammatic representation

32 Atlas of Histology for Medical Students

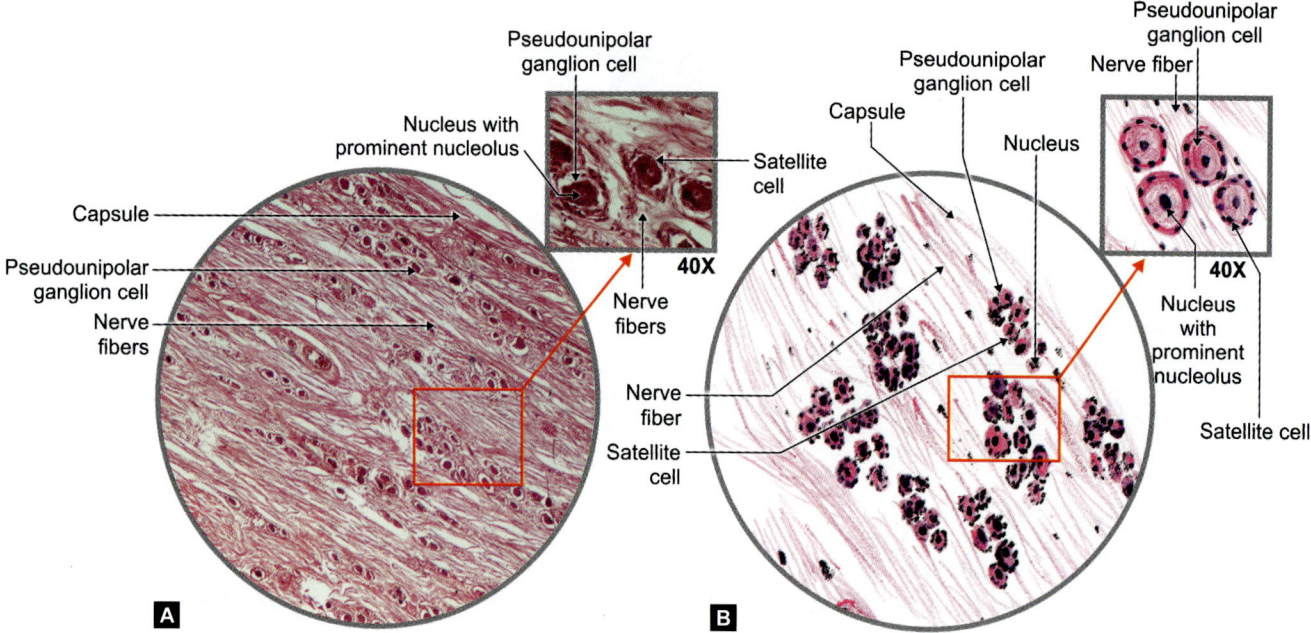

Figs 9.8A and B: (A) Microphotograph: Dorsal root ganglion (4X); (B) Diagrammatic representation

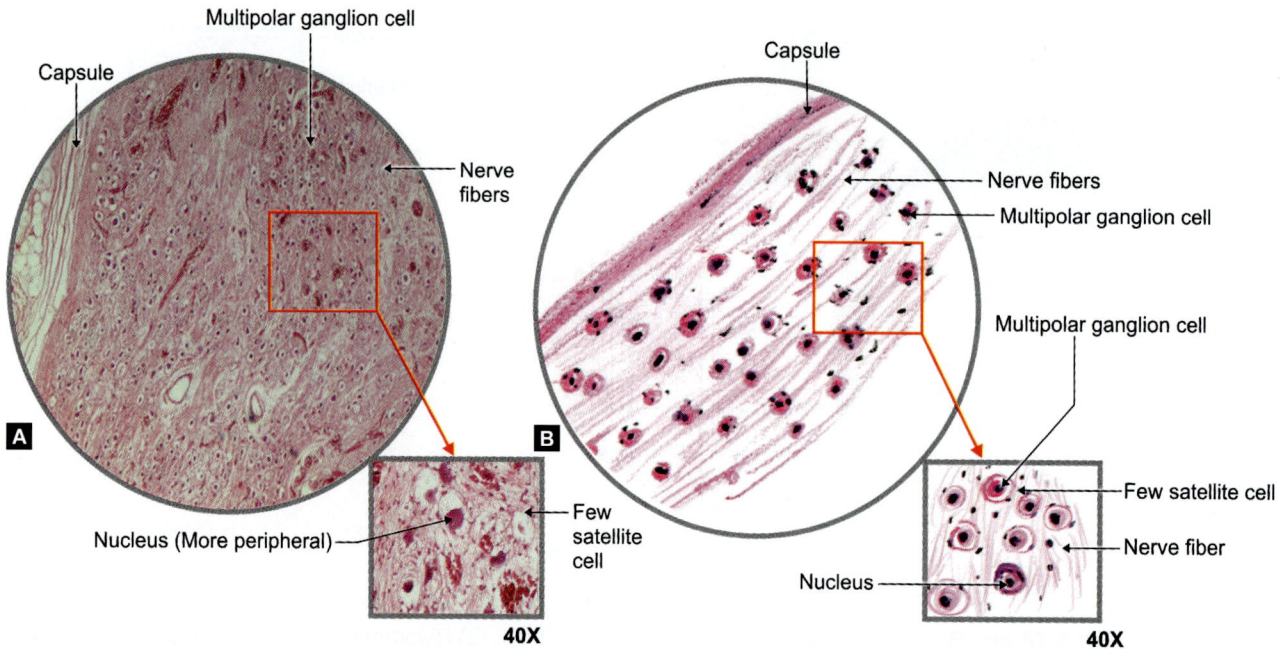

Figs 9.9A and B: (A) Microphotograph: Autonomic ganglion (4X); (B) Diagrammatic representation

CHAPTER 10

Cardiovascular System

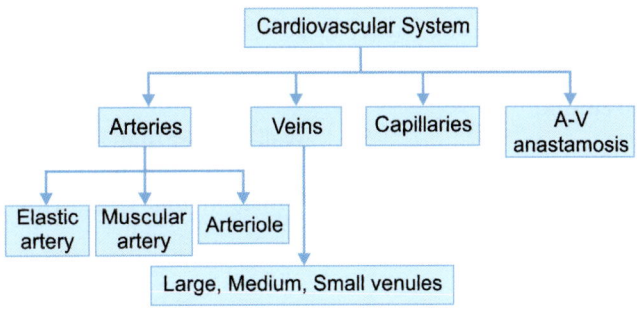

- A transport system to carry blood and lymph to and from the tissues of the body
- 2 Types of circulation:
  - Systemic: Conveys blood from heart to tissues and vice versa
  - Pulmonary: Conveys blood from heart to lungs and vice versa.

Three layers of wall of any blood vessel from lumen outwards are:
1. *Tunica intima*: Innermost layer
   Endothelium: Single layer of squamous epithelium
   Basal lamina of endothelium
   Lamina propria: Subendothelial layer
   Internal elastic membrane of concentric elastic fibers
2. *Tunica media*: Outside the intima layer
   Concentrically arranged smooth muscle cells
   Variable amount of elastin and reticular fibers, proteoglycans
   External elastic membrane
3. *Tunica adventitia*: Outermost layer
   Connective tissue: Longitudinally arranged collagen fibers, few elastin fibers
   Large vessels-Vasa vasorum (vessels in wall), nervi vascularis (autonomic nerves).

34 Atlas of Histology for Medical Students

Flow of blood in the systemic circulation

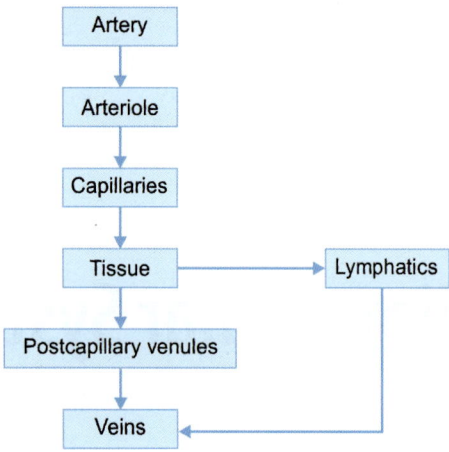

Artery Wall Thicker than Vein

Tunica media -2/3rd, Tunica Adventitia- 1/3rd
Elastic Artery (conducting vessels):
More elastic fibers in tunica media
Elastic membranes not prominent
E.g.: Large vessels like aorta, pulmonary trunk, brachiocephalic trunk, common carotid
Muscular Artery:
More smooth muscle fibers in tunica media
Elastic membranes prominent
E.g.: Smaller arteries.

Arteriole

Tunica media: 1–2 smooth muscle layers
Internal elastic membrane: May not be present
Tunica adventitia: Very thin.

Capillaries

Endothelial lining
Three types:

Continuous: Found in lung, central nervous system, muscle
Fenestrated: Found in endocrine glands, gallbladder, gastrointestinal tract.
Discontinuous/ sinusoidal: Irregular in shape, bigger in size, found in liver, spleen, bone marrow.

A-V Anastomosis

Found in skin of fingertips, nose, lips, erectile tissue of penis, clitoris.

Veins

Wall thinner than artery
Lumen is larger than the wall
Tunica media -1/3rd, Tunica adventitia- 2/3rd

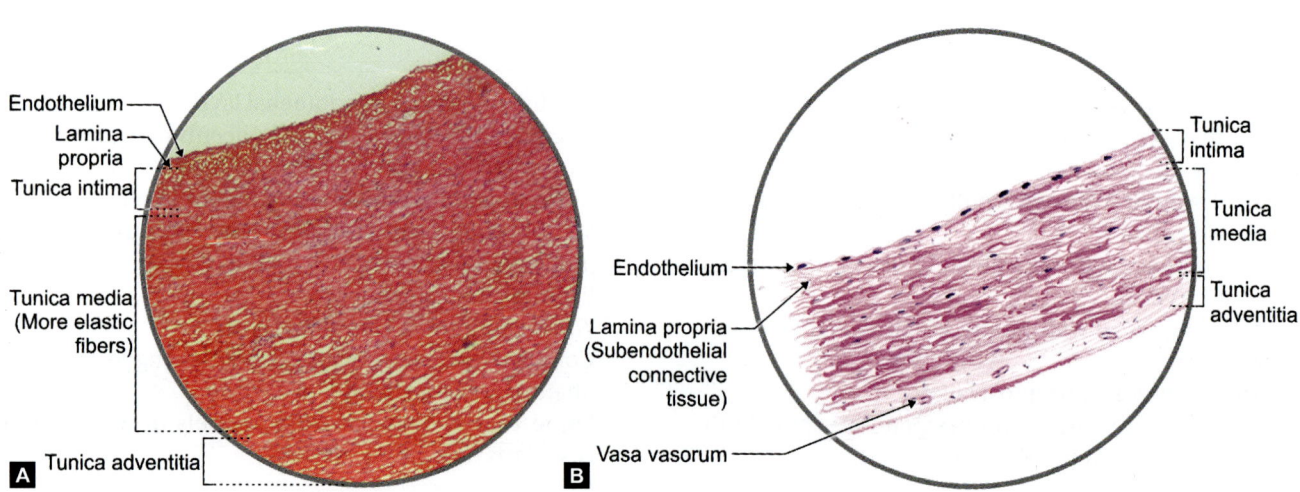

Figs 10.1A and B: (A) Microphotograph: Elastic artery (4X); (B) Diagrammatic representation

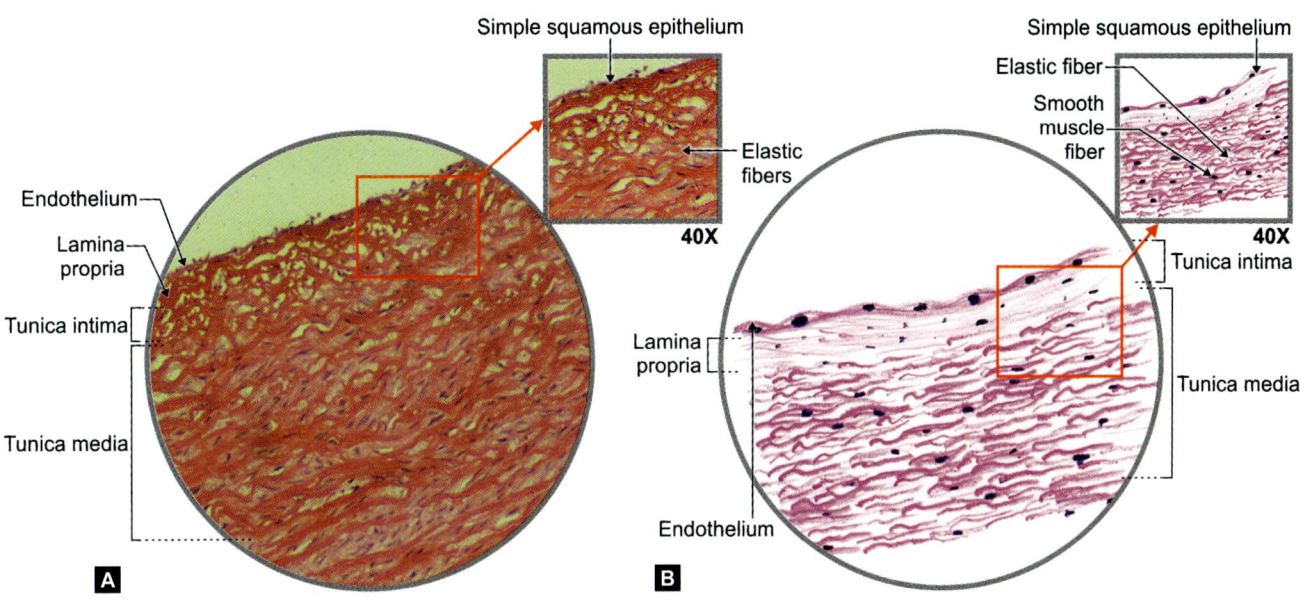

Figs 10.2A and B: (A) Microphotograph: Elastic artery (20X); (B) Diagrammatic representation

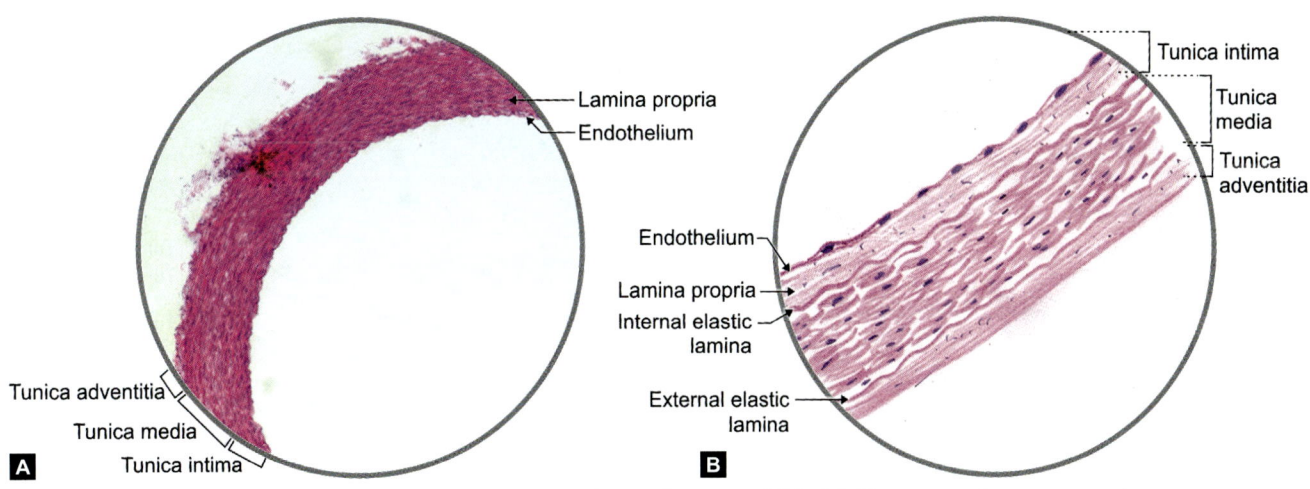

Figs 10.3A and B: (A) Microphotograph: Muscular artery (4X); (B) Diagrammatic representation

36 Atlas of Histology for Medical Students

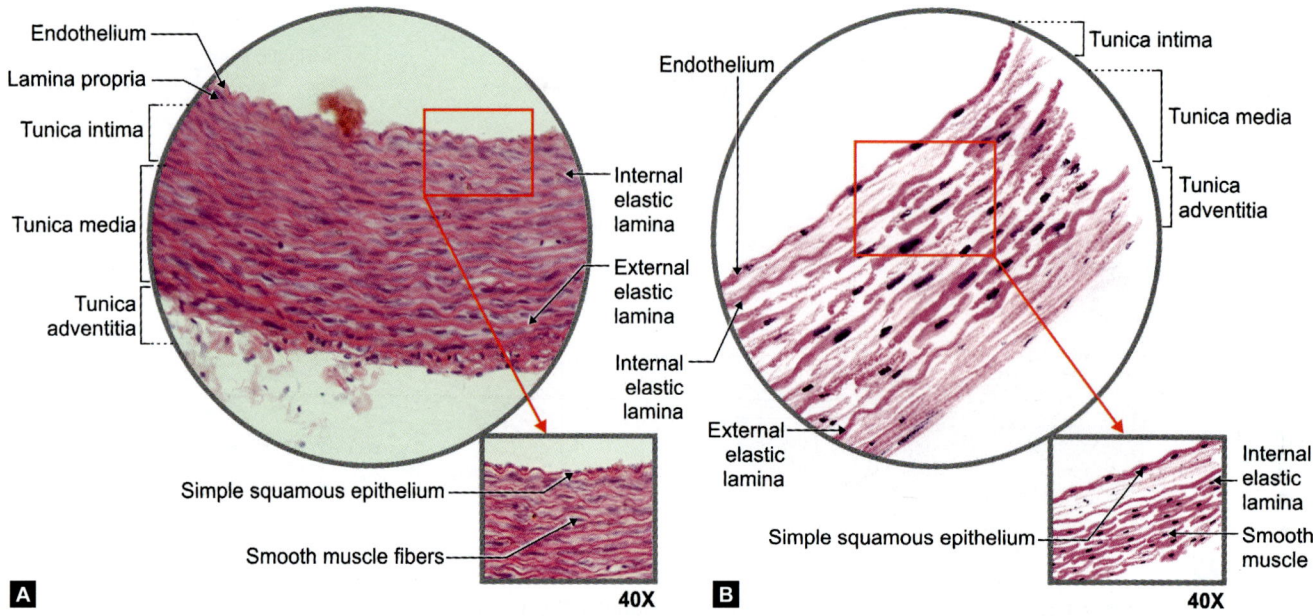

Figs 10.4A and B: (A) Microphotograph: Muscular artery (20X); (B) Diagrammatic representation

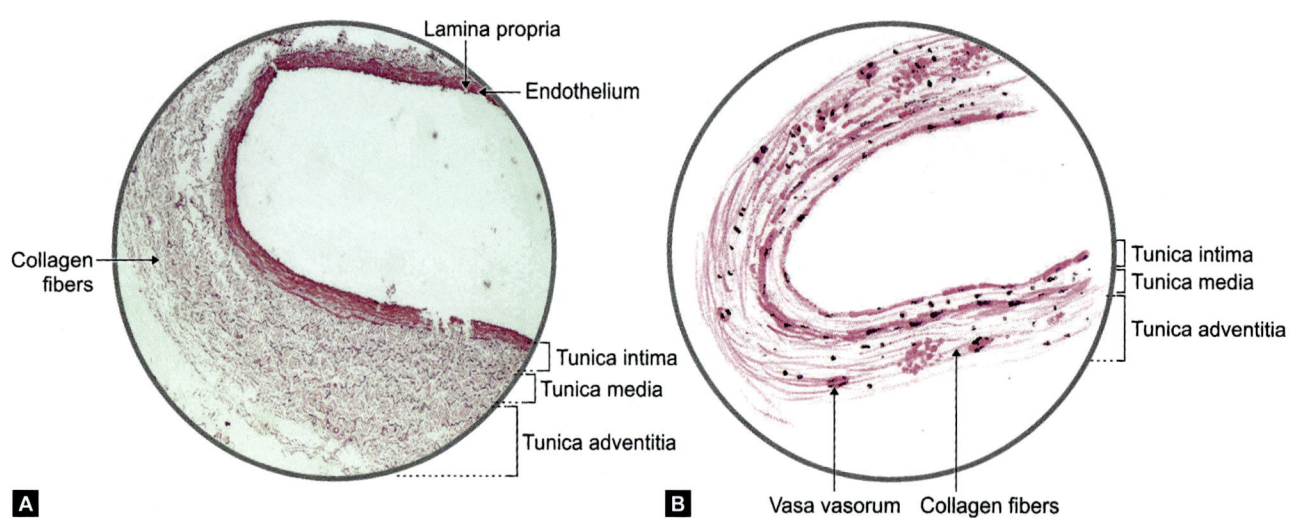

Figs 10.5A and B: (A) Microphotograph: Vein (4X); (B) Diagrammatic representation

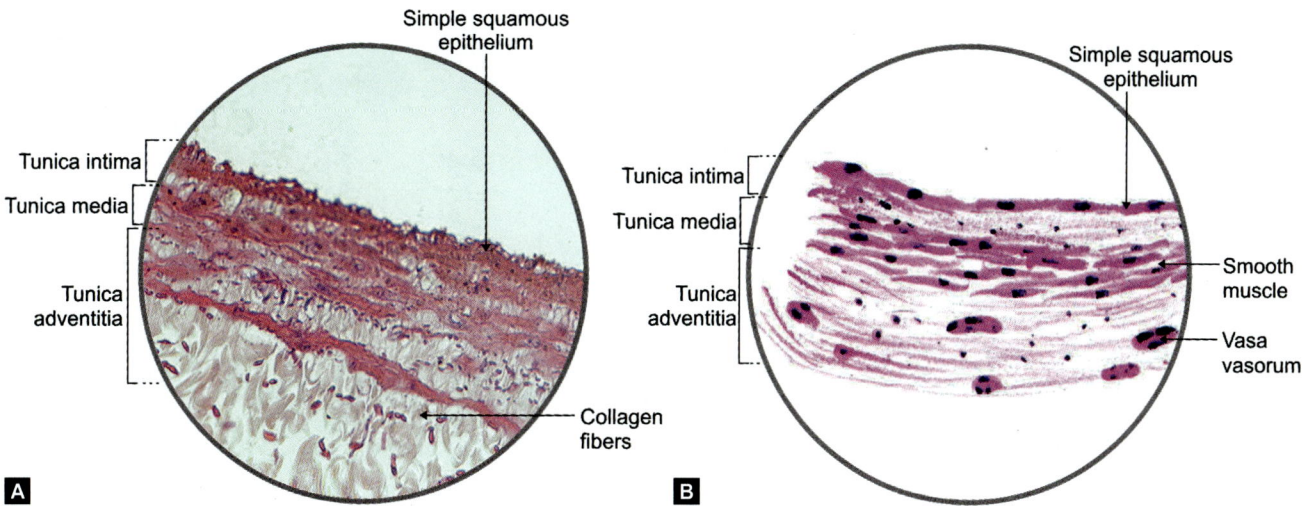

Figs 10.6A and B: (A) Microphotograph: Vein (20X); (B) Diagrammatic representation

CHAPTER 11

Lymphatic Tissue

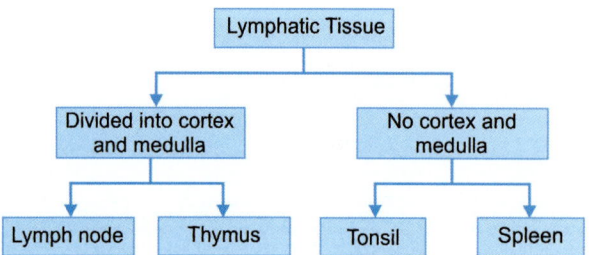

- Lymphatic system consists of various groups of cells, tissues and organs that are responsible for providing immunity to the body.
- Lymphatic vessels connect the lymph organs to the blood vascular system.

TABLE 11.1: Differentiating features of various lymphatic tissues

Feature	Lymph node	Thymus	Spleen	Tonsil
Capsule	Present	Present	Thick and lined by peritoneum	Capsule on pharyngeal side On oral side- Nonkeratinized stratified squamous epithelium
Subcapsular sinus	Present	Absent	Absent	Absent
Division into cortex and medulla	Present	Continuous medulla (incomplete septa)	Absent	Absent
Lymph follicles with germinal center	Present	Absent	Present with eccentrically placed central arteriole	Present
Medulla	Medullary cords	Hassal's corpuscles present	No medulla, Parenchyma divided into red and white pulp	Absent
Trabeculae	Thin all over	Only in peripheral or cortical part	Abundant thick with blood vessels	Occasional, thin

Lymphatic Tissue **39**

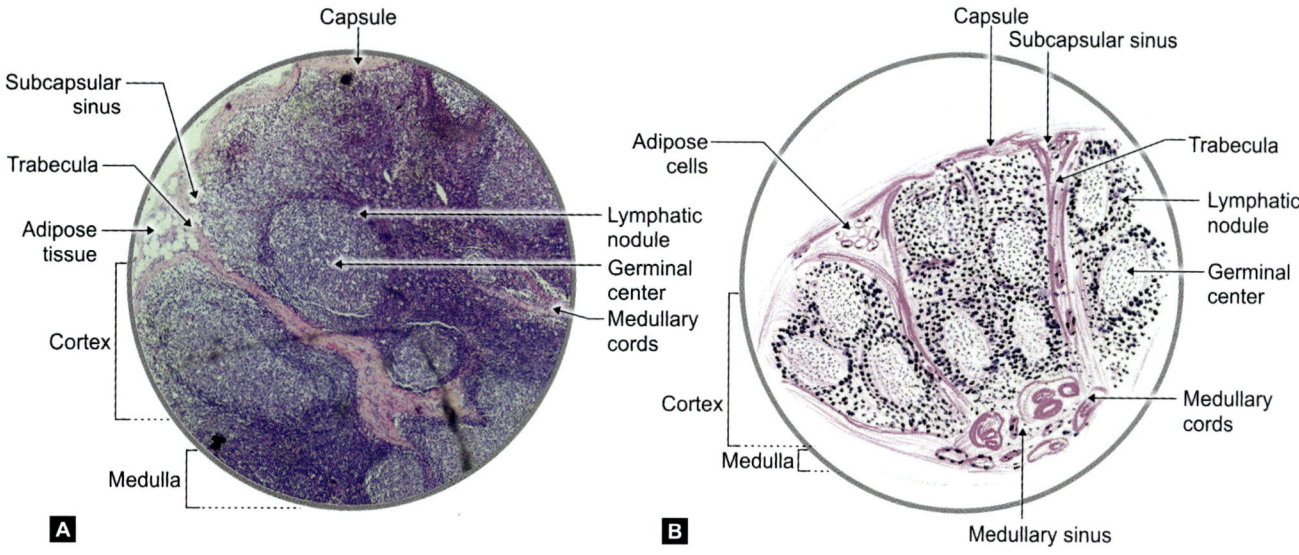

Figs 11.1A and B: (A) Microphotograph: Lymph node (4X); (B) Diagrammatic representation

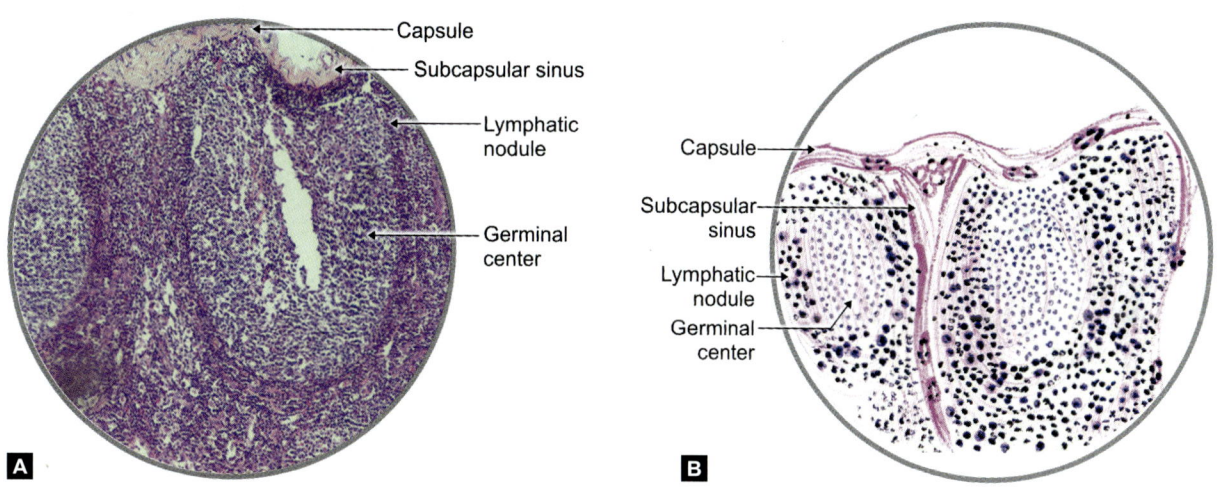

Figs 11.2A and B: (A) Microphotograph: Lymph node (20X); (B) Diagrammatic representation

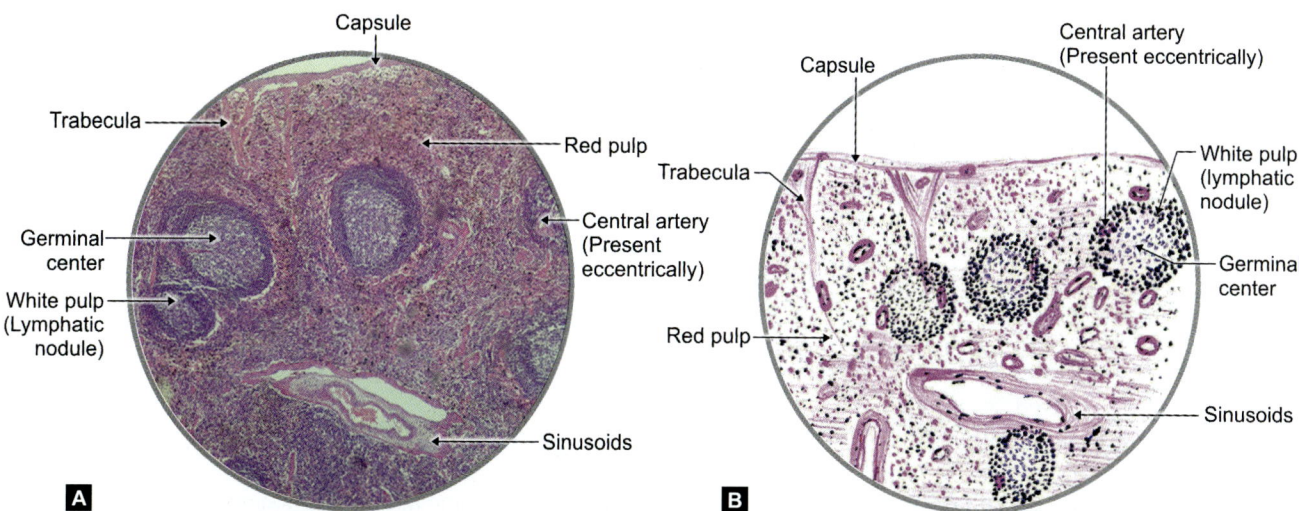

Figs 11.3A and B: (A) Microphotograph: Spleen (4X); (B) Diagrammatic representation

40 Atlas of Histology for Medical Students

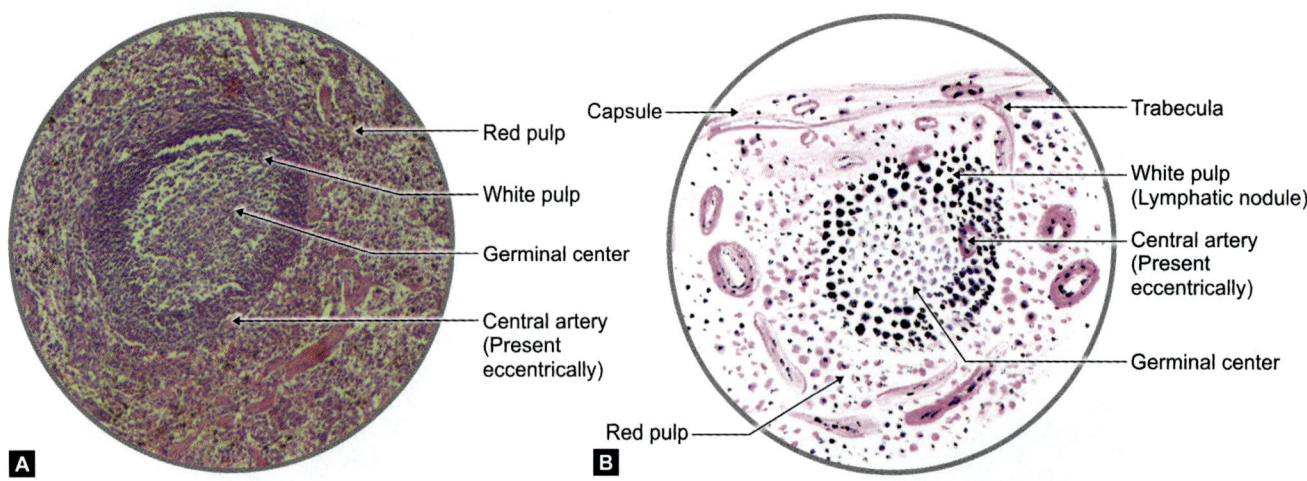

Figs 11.4A and B: (A) Microphotograph: Spleen (20X); (B) Diagrammatic representation

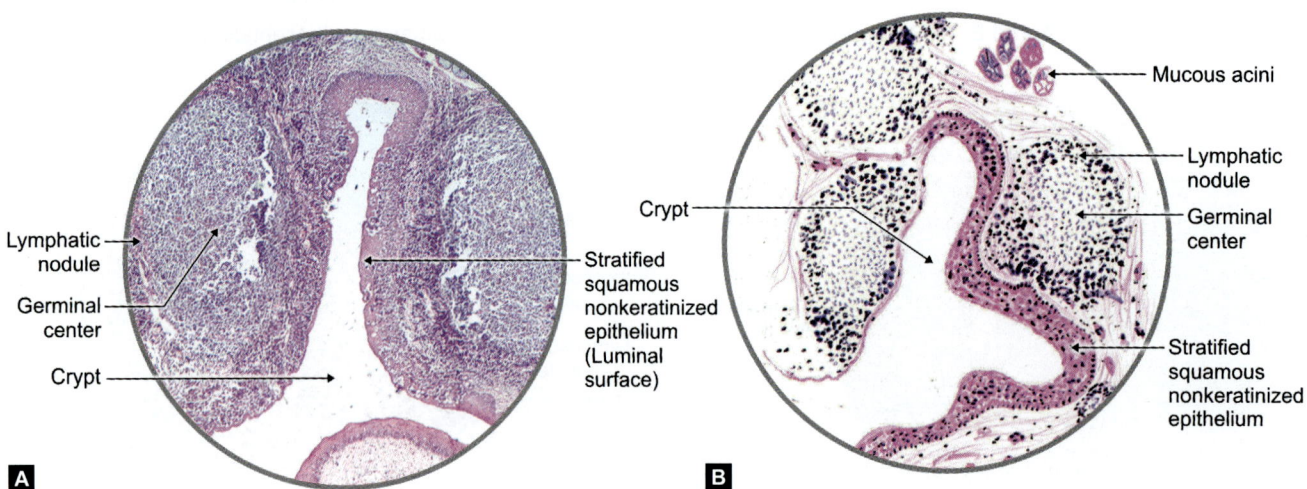

Figs 11.5A and B: (A) Microphotograph: Tonsil (4X); (B) Diagrammatic representation

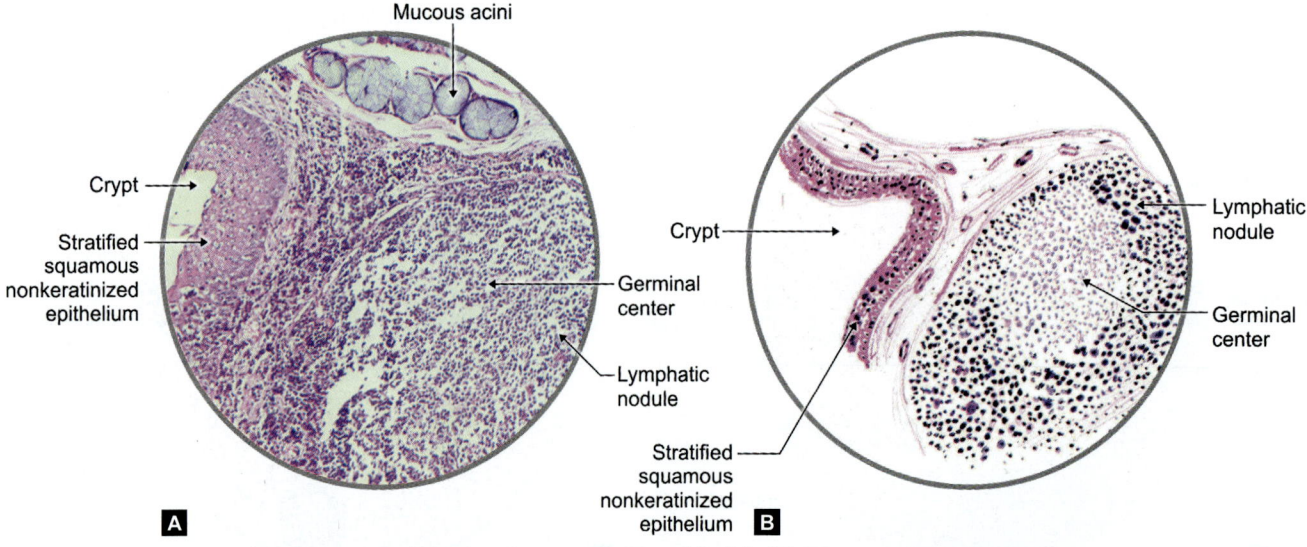

Figs 11.6A and B: (A) Microphotograph: Tonsil (20X); (B) Diagrammatic representation

Lymphatic Tissue **41**

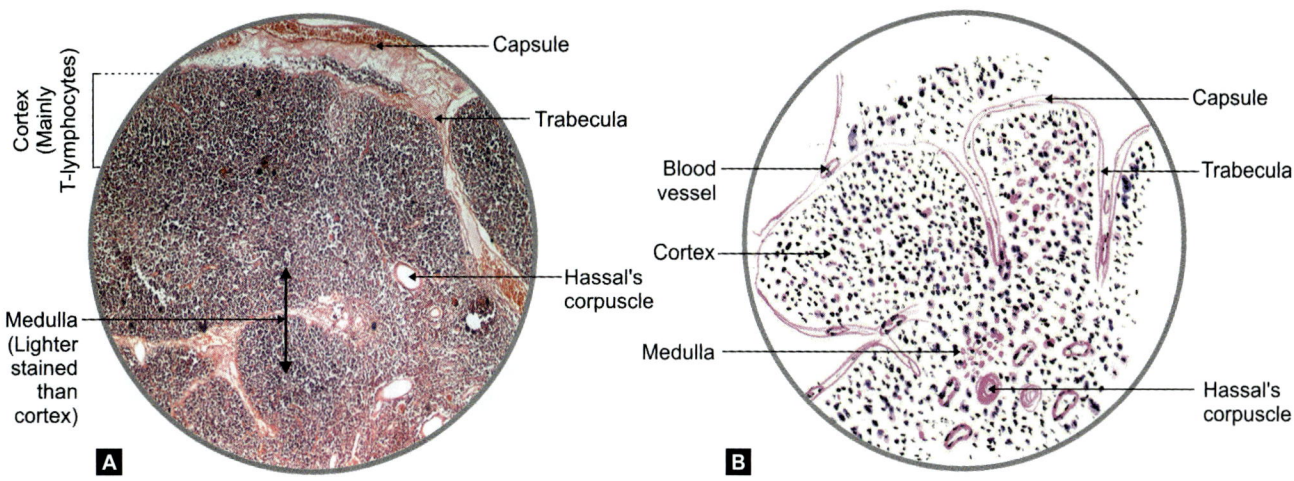

Figs 11.7A and B: (A) Microphotograph: Thymus (4X); (B) Diagrammatic representation

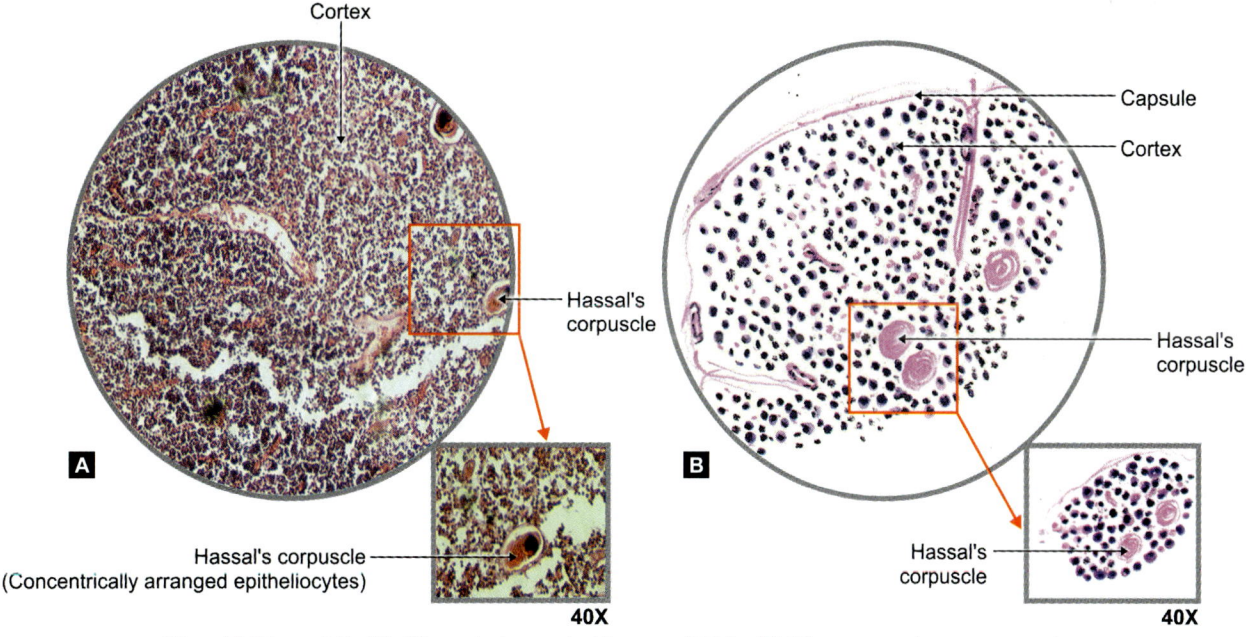

Figs 11.8A and B: (A) Microphotograph: Thymus (20X); (B) Diagrammatic representation

CHAPTER 12

Integumentary System

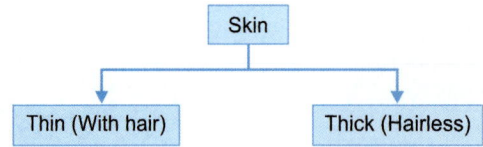

- Skin forms outer covering of body
- Largest organ (15-20% of total mass)
- First mechanical barrier against antigens
- Endocrine function
- Gives 1st sensory information from external environment
- Maintains homeostasis
- Excretion through secretions of glands present in epidermis

LAYERS OF SKIN

Epidermis

- *Epithelium:* Keratinized stratified squamous, regenerating with epidermal (rete) ridges:
    - Gives rise to nails, hair, sebaceous and sweat glands.

From Deepest to Superficial

- *Stratum basale (germinativum):* Basal layer of mitotically active (stem cell) cuboidal to low coloumnar cells (basophilic)
- *Stratum spinosum:* Prickle cell appearance due to short processes between cells (cells shrink during processing of tissue-so look spinous)
- *Stratum granulosum:* Many granules in cytoplasm of cells (darkly stained, keratohyalin granules)
- *Stratum lucidum:* Glass-like (refractile) appearance of cells
- *Stratum corneum:* Keratinized (dead) cells, keratin filaments without nuclei
- *Keratin:* Lipid layer, water barrier.

TABLE 12.1: Differentiating features between thick skin and thin skin

Features	Thick skin	Thin skin
Thickness	Epidermis thicker, keratin layer thicker	Thin
Stratum lucidum and corneum	Present	Absent
Hair	Hairless	Hair follicles
Dermis	Papillae are longer, closely placed	Papillae further placed and smaller
Location	Places of more abrasion—palms, soles	Rest of the body

Dermis

- Dense connective tissue
- Main thickness of the skin
- Support and strength to tissue

- *Dermal papillae:* Finger-like connective tissue protrusions.

Hypodermis

- Adipose tissue (superficial fascia)

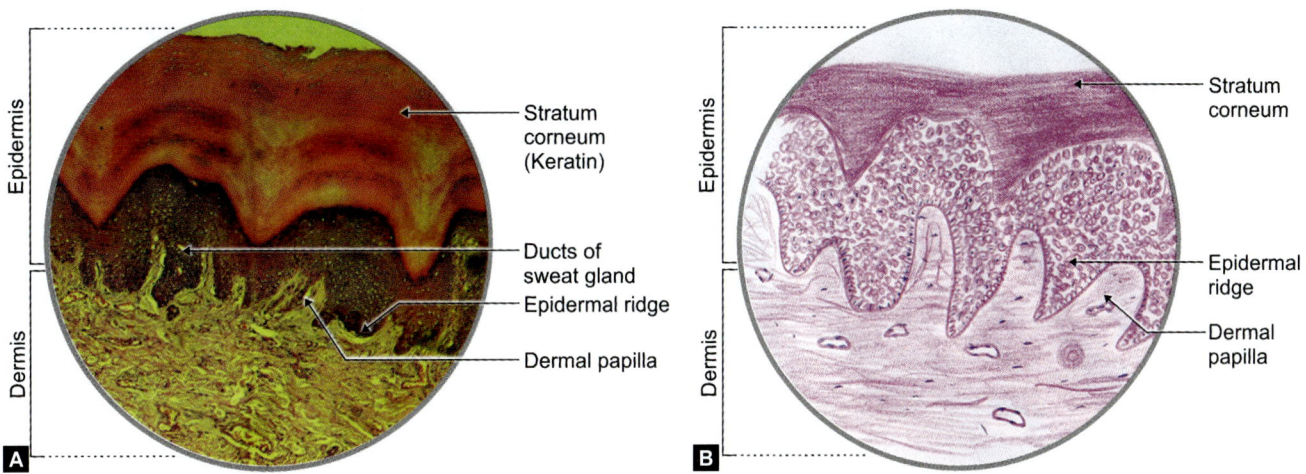

Figs 12.1A and B: (A) Microphotograph: Thick skin (4X); (B) Diagrammatic representation

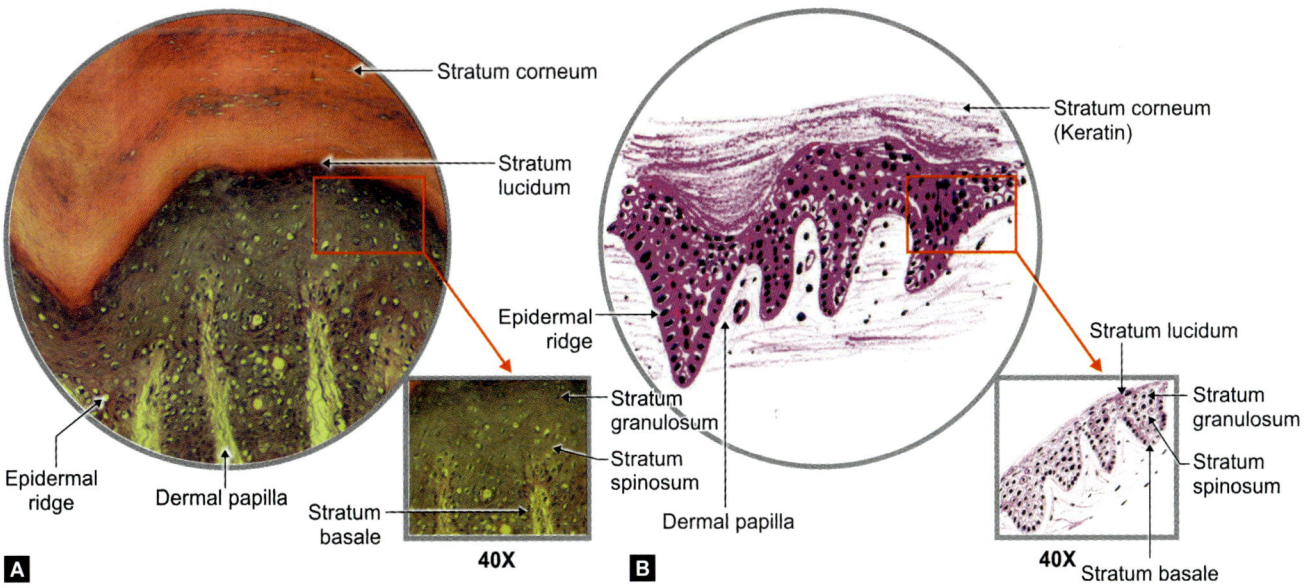

Figs 12.2A and B: (A) Microphotograph: Thick skin (20X); (B) Diagrammatic representation

44 Atlas of Histology for Medical Students

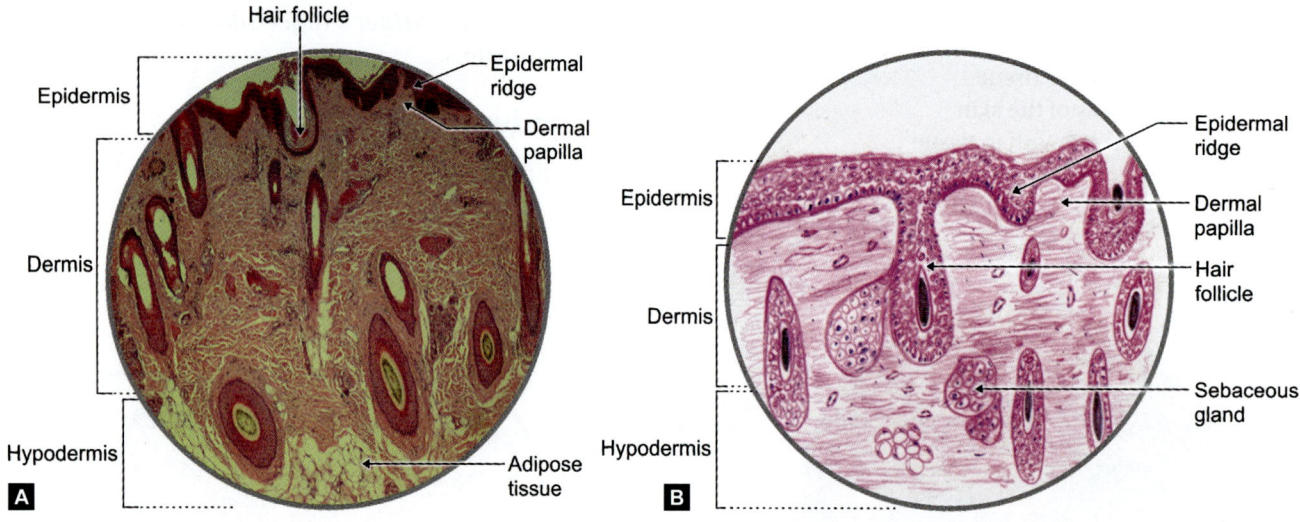

Figs 12.3A and B: (A) Microphotograph: Thin skin (4X); (B) Diagrammatic representation

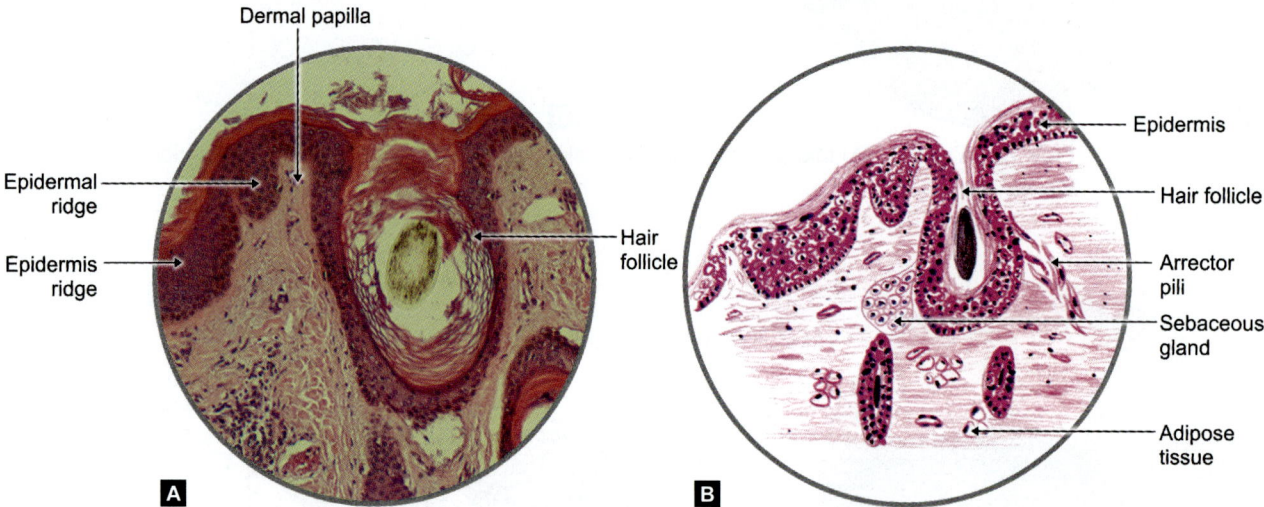

Figs 12.4A and B: (A) Microphotograph: Thin skin (20X); (B) Diagrammatic representation

CHAPTER 13

Digestive System

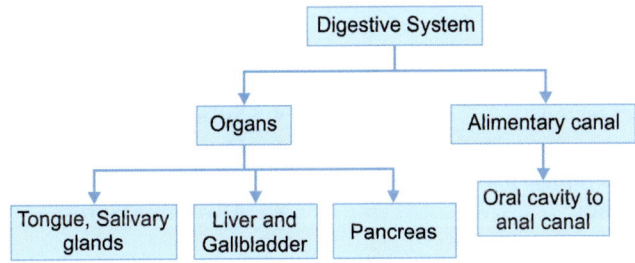

Tongue: Ventral and dorsal surfaces
- Epithelium: Ventral surface- oral mucosa- stratified squamous non keratinized epithelium
- Dorsal surface- with papillae- filiform, fungiform, circumvallate with taste buds
- Lamina propria
- Core of striated muscle: Running in 3 different planes
- Salivary glands: Both mucous and serous.

SALIVARY GLANDS

- Exocrine glands (give secretions via ducts)
- Consists of:
  - Stroma—
    - Capsule (connective tissue), septa
    - Blood vessels
  - Parenchyma—
    - Acini— (Serous/ Mucous) *[See Chapter 4]*
    - Myoepithelial cells
  - Ducts
- Secrete saliva
- Major: Parotid, sublingual, submandibular.
- Minor: In oral cavity.

LIVER

- Largest gland of the body
- Glisson's capsule- Connective tissue
- Stroma
  - Consists of connective tissue
  - Divides parenchyma into hepatic lobules (basic structural unit of liver)
  - Blood vessels are carried through them

- Parenchyma
  - Basic cell- Hepatocyte (polyhedral in shape)
  - Basic structural unit of liver- Hepatic lobule- hexagonal in shape.

Hepatic Lobule

- Hepatocyte arranged in anastomosing plates radiating from a central point where central vein is present
- Hepatic (fenestrated) sinusoids present between plates of hepatocytes (lined by endothelium and Kupffer cells)
- Space of Disse: Space between hepatocytes and endothelium of sinusoids.

At Six Angles of Hepatic Lobule

- Tributary of portal vein
- A branch of hepatic artery
- A branch of bile duct
- Occasionally lymphatic vessel.

PANCREAS

- Present in the concavity of duodenum
- Has 4 parts: - Head, Neck, Body, Tail
- Histologically has two parts—
  - Exocrine part with duct system
    - Serous glands (acini— pyramidal cells with rounded nuclei at base, apical part—eosinophilic, basal part—basophilic)
    - Duct system with intercalated ducts lined by centroacinar cells (centrally placed nucleus, pale cytoplasm)
  - Islets of Langerhans: Endocrine part with blood vessels
    - Irregular cords of Polyhedral cells (alpha, beta, delta)
    - Capillaries interspersed in between the cells.

GALLBLADDER

- Histologically three layers
- From deep to superficial:
  - Mucosa: Numerous folds with brush border simple columnar epithelium *(no goblet cells)*
  - ***Submucosa- absent***
  - Muscularis externa: Smooth muscle fibers arranged in different planes
  - Serosa: Covered by peritoneum.

From Esophagus to Large Intestine

Histologically four layers:

- Mucosa: Epithelium, Lamina propria, Muscularis mucosa
- Submucosa: Dense irregular connective tissue
- Muscularis externa: Generally consists of 2 layers of smooth muscle
- Adventitia/Serosa.

TABLE 13.1: Differentiating features between various parts of digestive system

		Esophagus	Stomach	Small intestine	Large intestine
Mucosa	Epithelium	Nonkeratinized stratified squamous	Simple columnar with gastric glands (*Parietal/Oxyntic, Zymogen/Chief cells*)	Columnar epithelium with Microvilli (Striated border)	Columnar epithelium with *goblet cells (1/3rd)*
	Villi	--	--	Present	--
	Lamina propria	Connective tissue	Gastric glands	*Crypts of Lieberkuhn (intestinal glands/crypts)*	Intestinal glands
	Muscularis mucosa	+	+	+	+
Submucosa		Rugae—temporary folds Mucous secreting esophageal glands	Present	*Plicae circularis/ Valves of Kerckring- permanent folds* Submucous glands of Brunner--- duodenum Peyer's patches-- ileum	Present
Muscularis externa		Upper 1/3rd-striated Middle 1/3rd- mixed Lower 1/3rd- smooth	Three layers—Inner oblique, middle circular, outer longitudinal	Two layers—Inner circular, outer longitudinal	Two layers—Inner circular, outer longitudinal Longitudinal— three thick bands of muscle called *taenia coli*
Serosa/Adventitia		Present	Present	Present	Present

Digestive System

TABLE 13.2: Differentiating features between various parts of small intestine

		Duodenum	Jejunum	Ileum
Mucosa	Epithelium	Simple columnar with goblet cells Microvilli (Striated border)	Simple columnar with goblet cells Microvilli (Striated border) Greater mucosal folds	Simple columnar with goblet cells Microvilli (Striated border)
	Lamina propria	Villi Spatulate, broad	Villi Tongue shaped Larger	Villi Few, thin, finger like
Submucosa	Crypts of Liberkuhn (Plica circularis)	Present	Present Larger and more closely set	Present Smaller and sparse
	Brunners glands (mucous acini)	Present	–	–
	Peyer's patches	–	–	Present

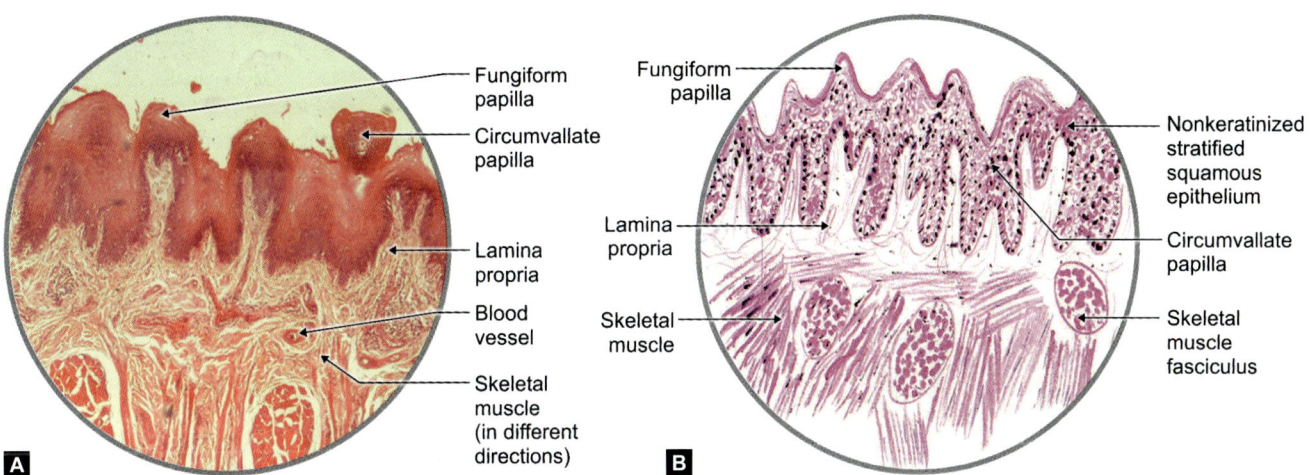

Figs 13.1A and B: (A) Microphotograph: Tongue (10X); (B) Diagrammatic representation

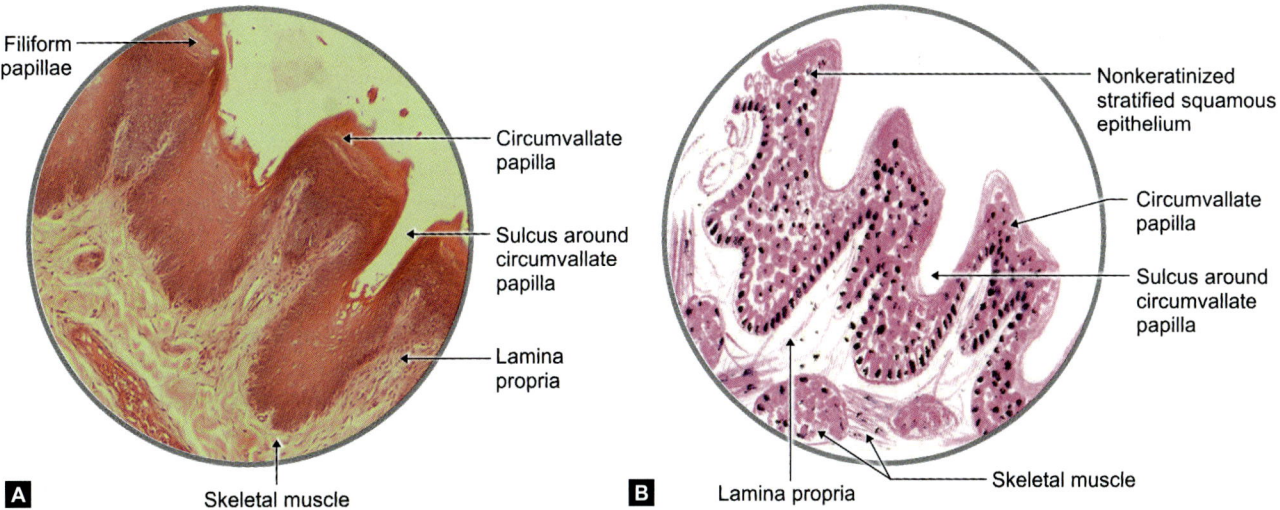

Figs 13.2A and B: (A) Microphotograph: Tongue (20X); (B) Diagrammatic representation

48 Atlas of Histology for Medical Students

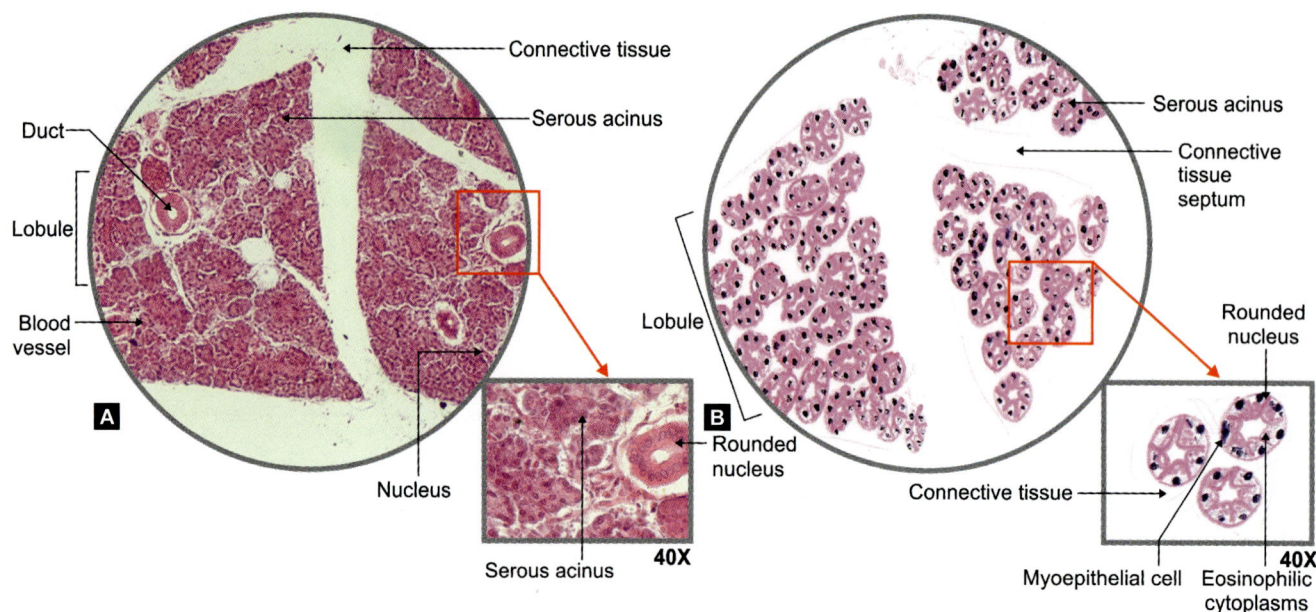

Figs 13.3A and B: (A) Microphotograph: Parotid gland (10X); (B) Diagrammatic representation

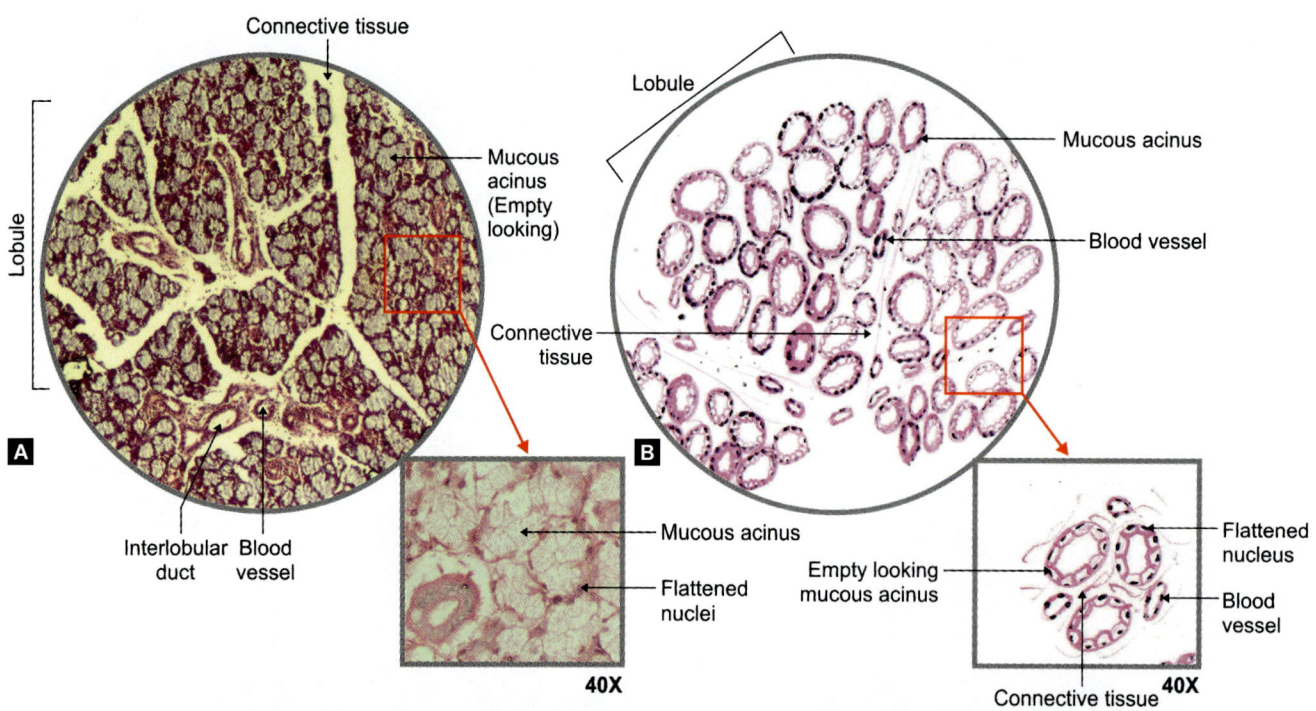

Figs 13.4A and B: (A) Microphotograph: Sublingual gland (10X); (B) Diagrammatic representation

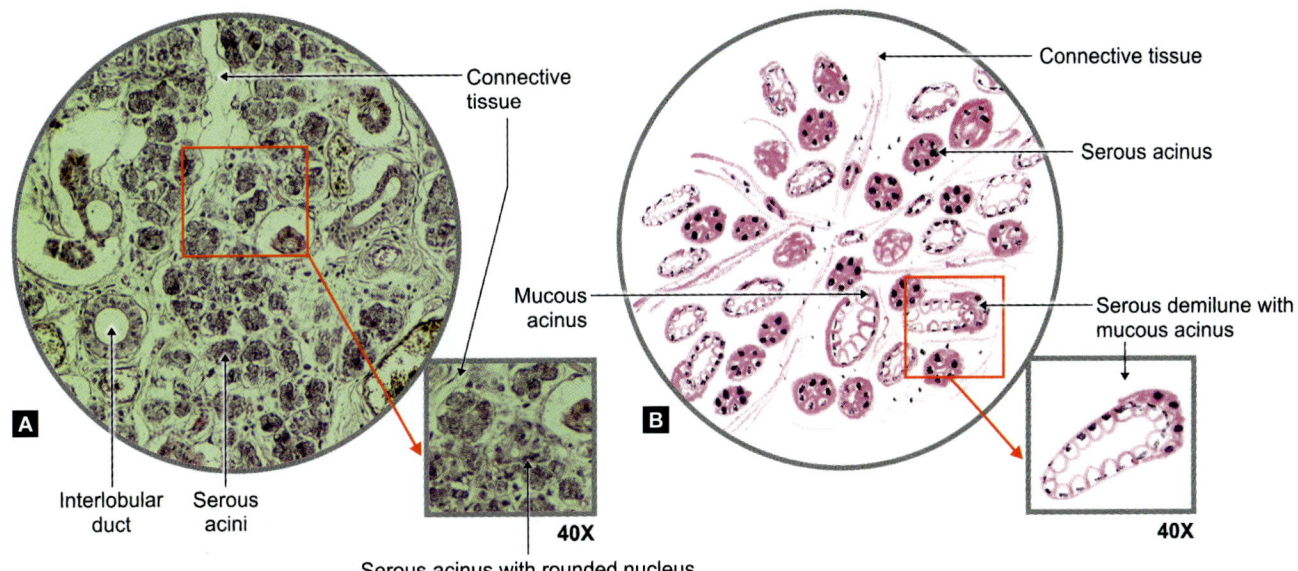

Figs 13.5A and B: (A) Microphotograph: Submandibular gland (10X); (B) Diagrammatic representation

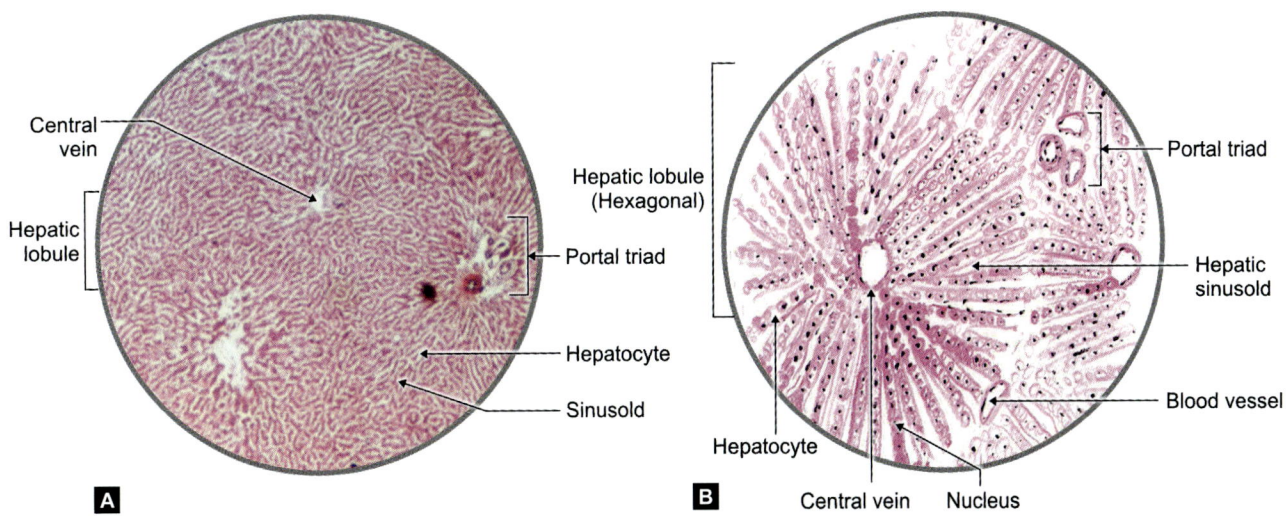

Figs 13.6A and B: (A) Microphotograph: Liver (4X); (B) Diagrammatic representation

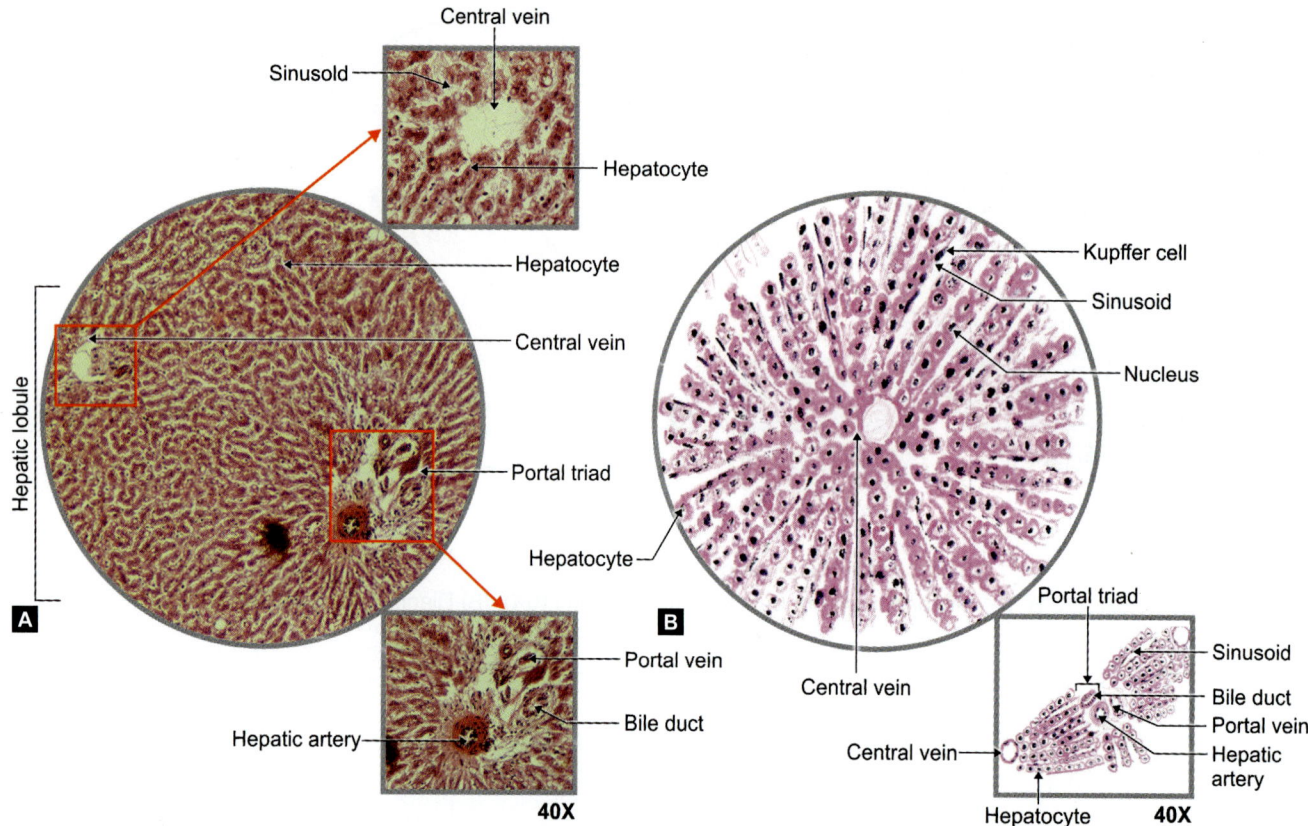

Figs 13.7A and B: (A) Microphotograph: Liver (20X); (B) Diagrammatic representation

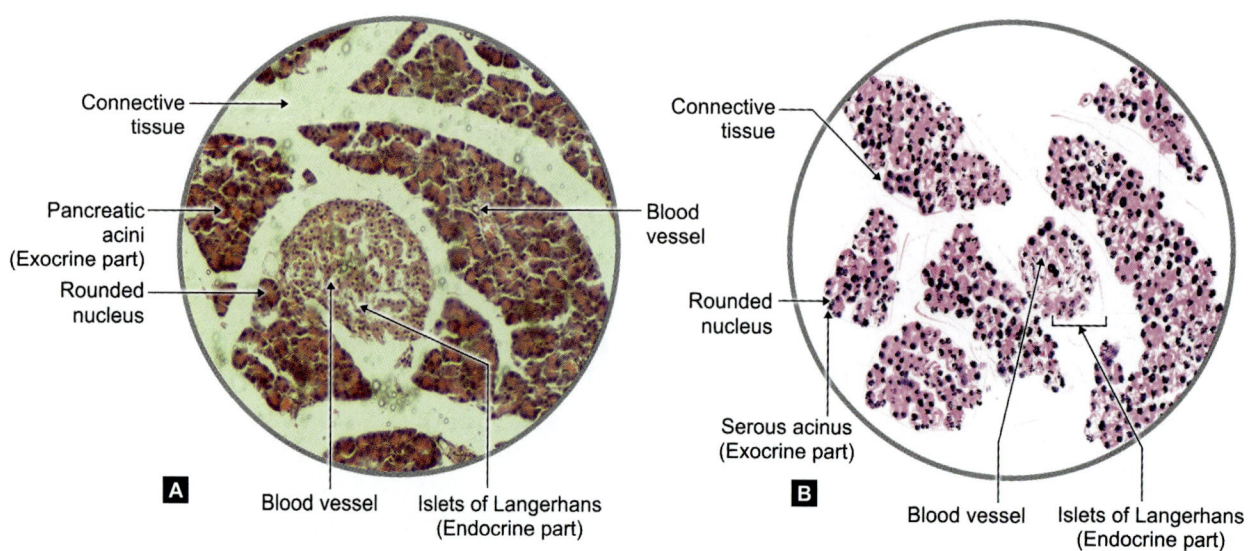

Figs 13.8A and B: (A) Microphotograph: Pancreas (4X); (B) Diagrammatic representation

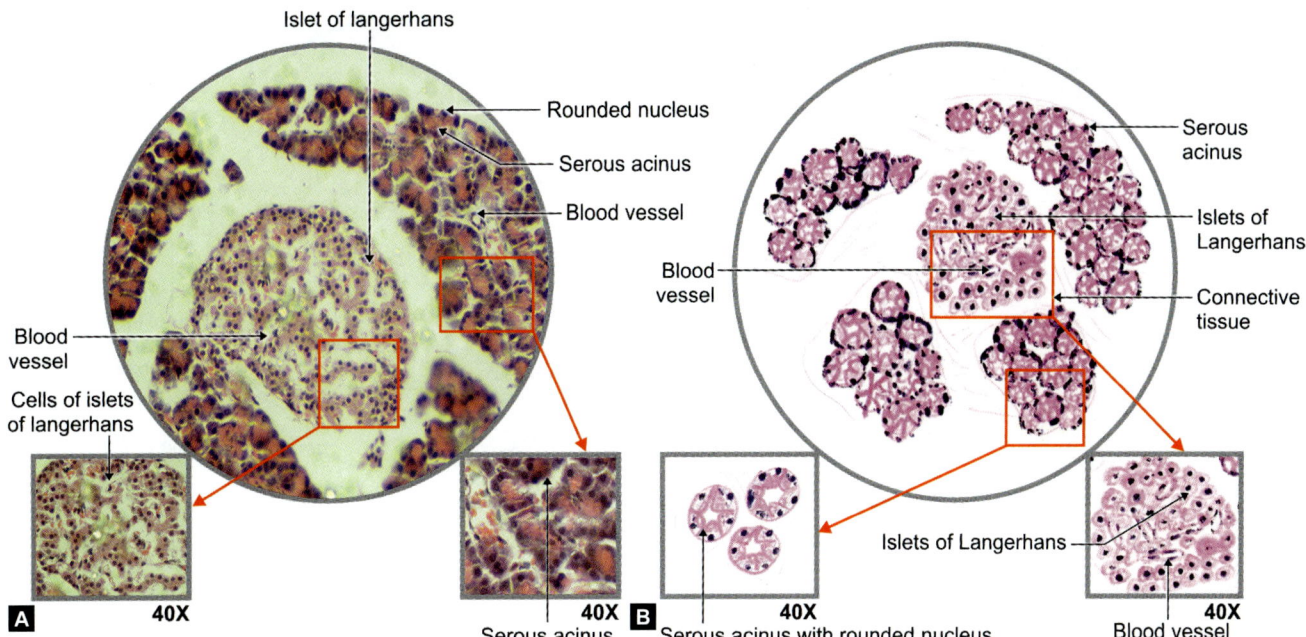

Figs 13.9A and B: (A) Microphotograph: Pancreas (20X); (B) Diagrammatic representation

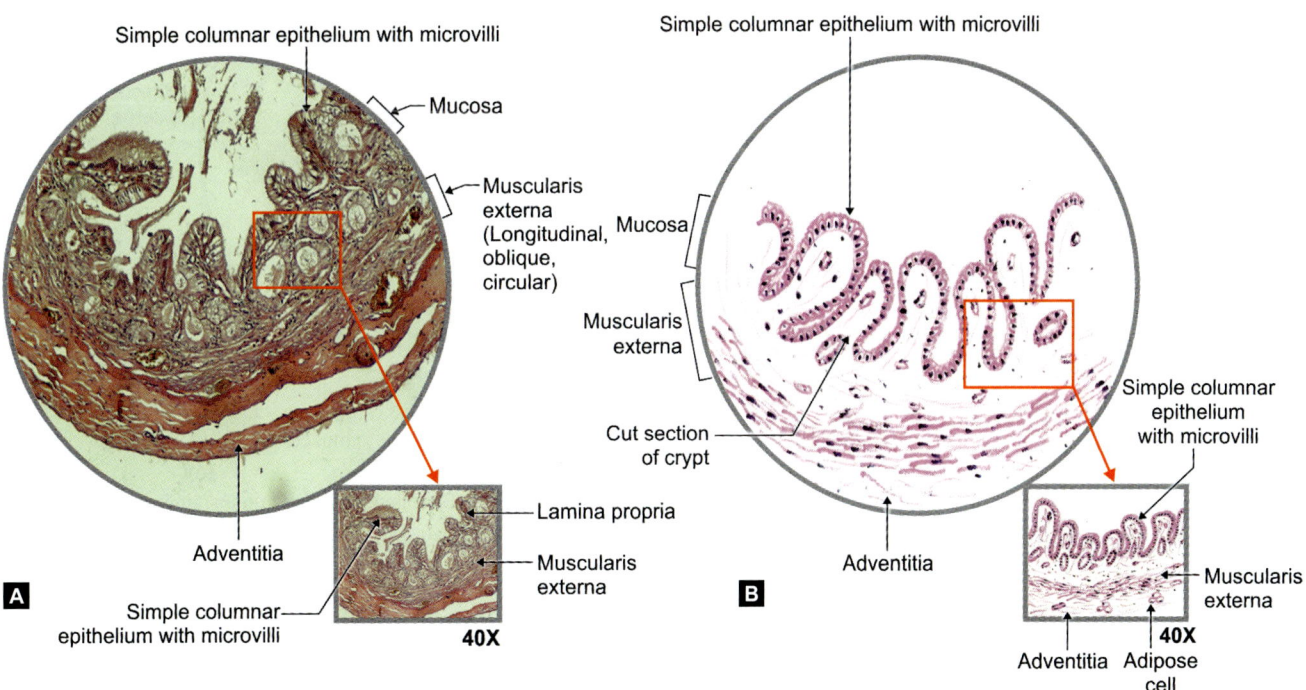

Figs 13.10A and B: (A) Microphotograph: Gallbladder (4X); (B) Diagrammatic representation

52 Atlas of Histology for Medical Students

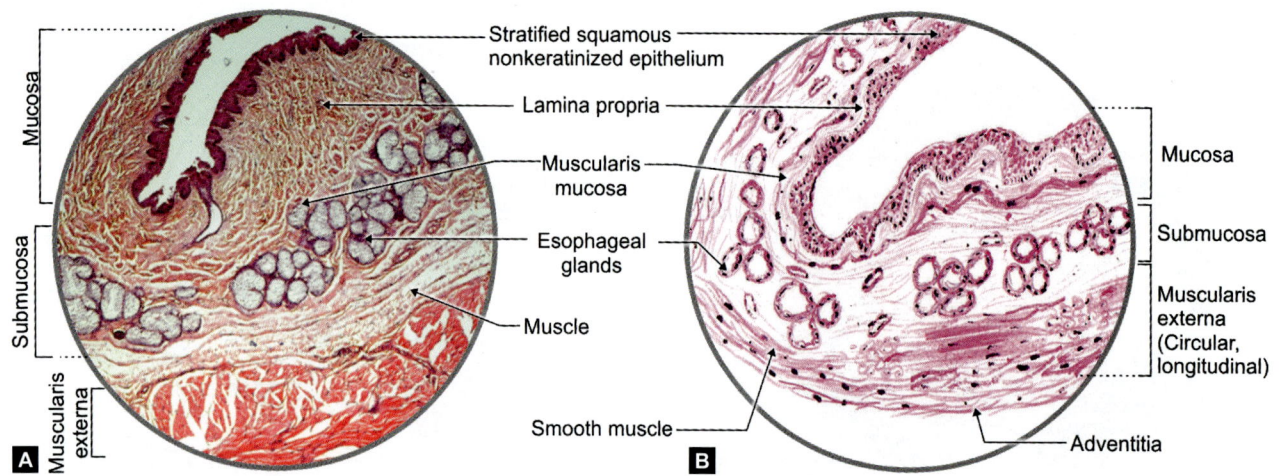

Figs 13.11A and B: (A) Microphotograph: Esophagus (4X); (B) Diagrammatic representation

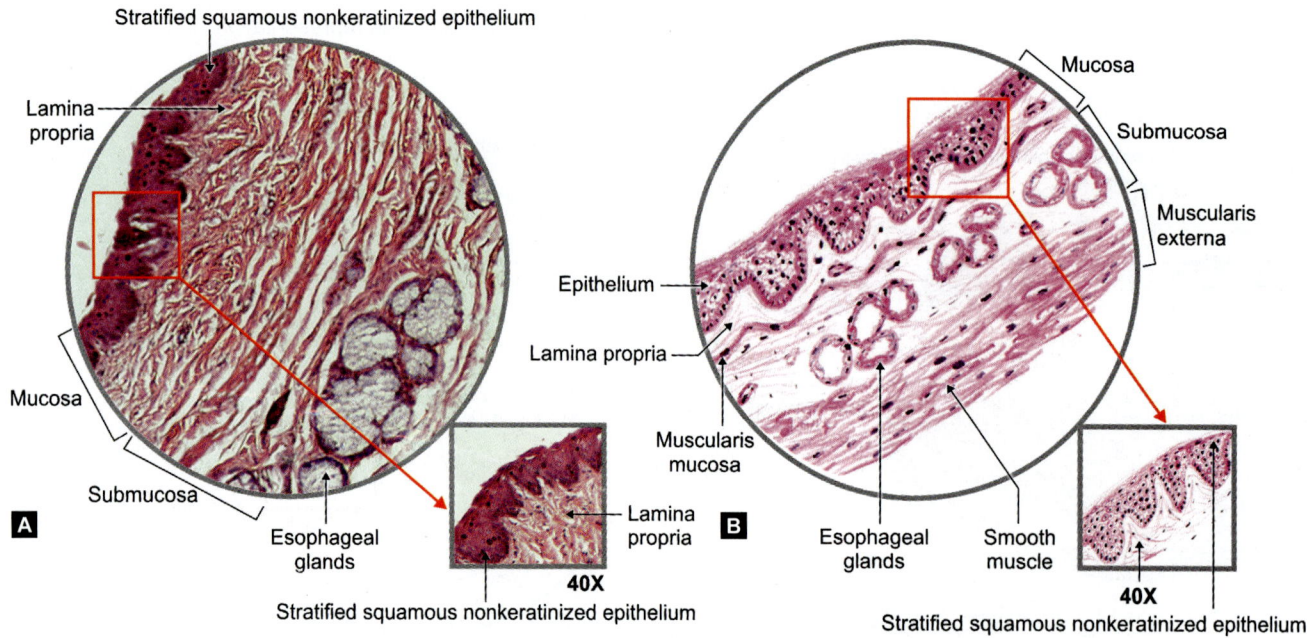

Figs 13.12A and B: (A) Microphotograph: Esophagus (20X); (B) Diagrammatic representation

Digestive System

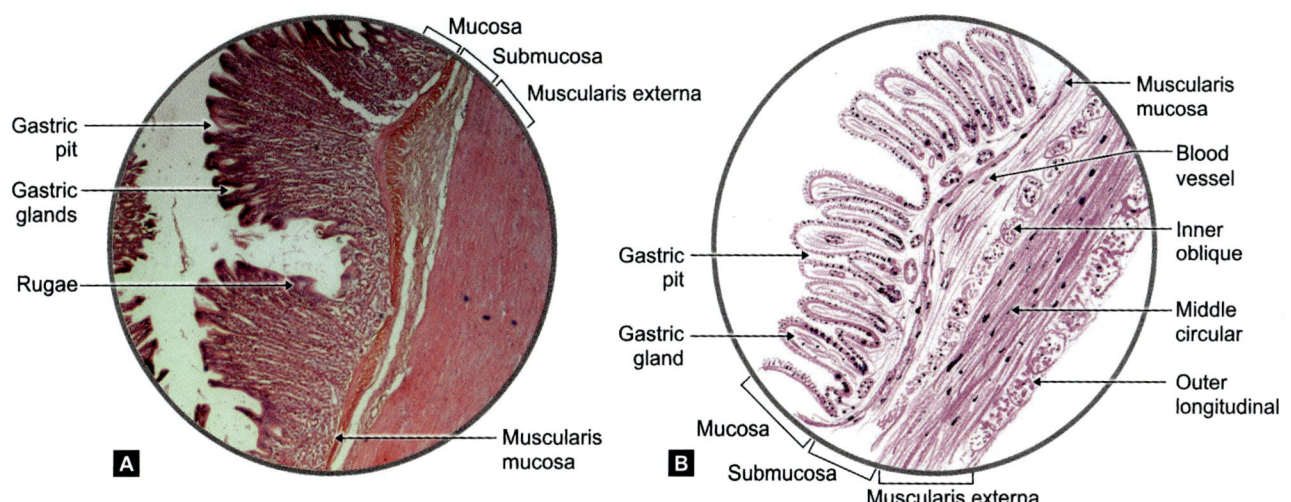

Figs 13.13A and B: (A) Microphotograph: Stomach (Fundus)(4X); (B) Diagrammatic representation

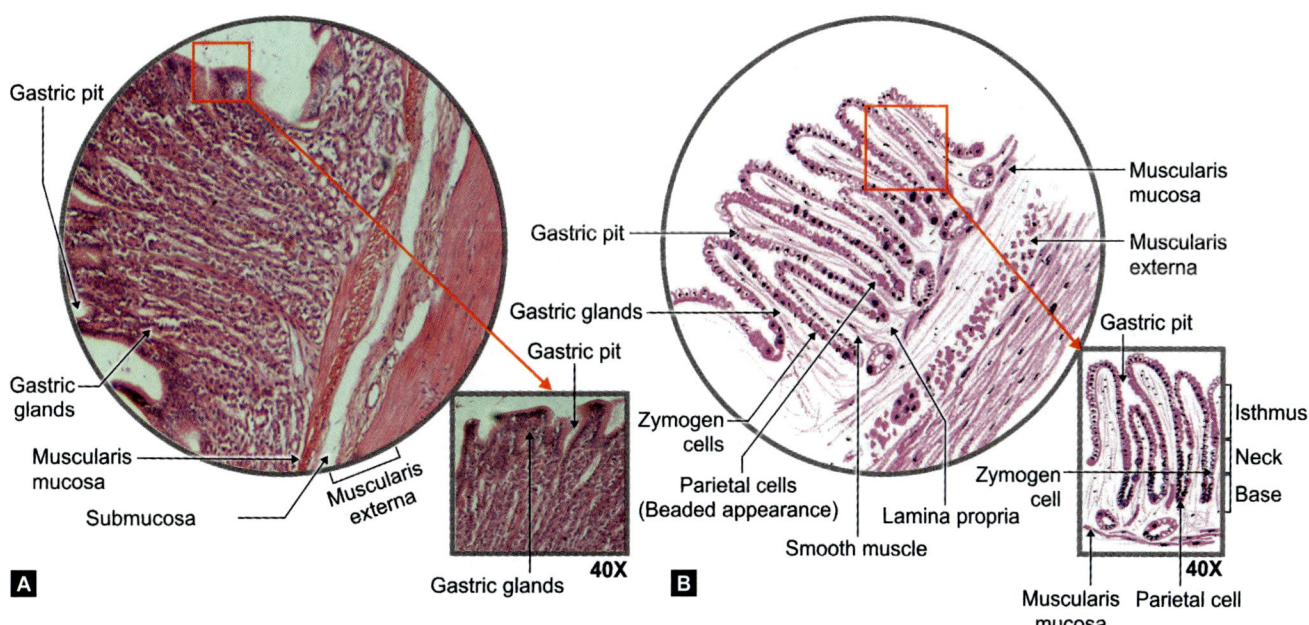

Figs 13.14A and B: (A) Microphotograph: Stomach (Fundus)(20X); (B) Diagrammatic representation

54 Atlas of Histology for Medical Students

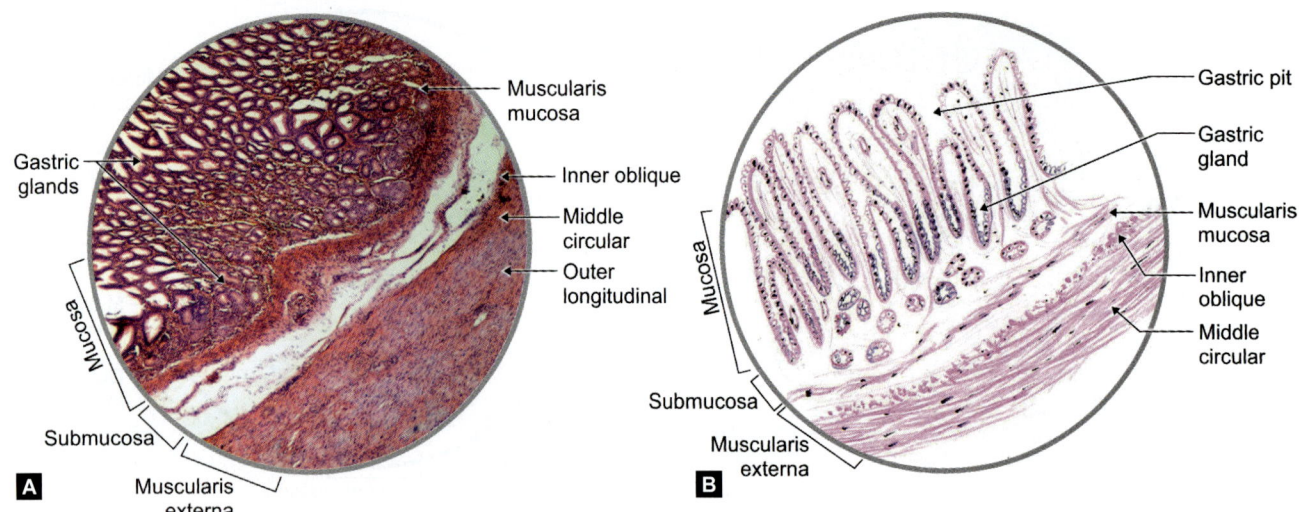

Figs 13.15A and B: (A) Microphotograph: Stomach (Pyloric)(20X); (B) Diagrammatic representation

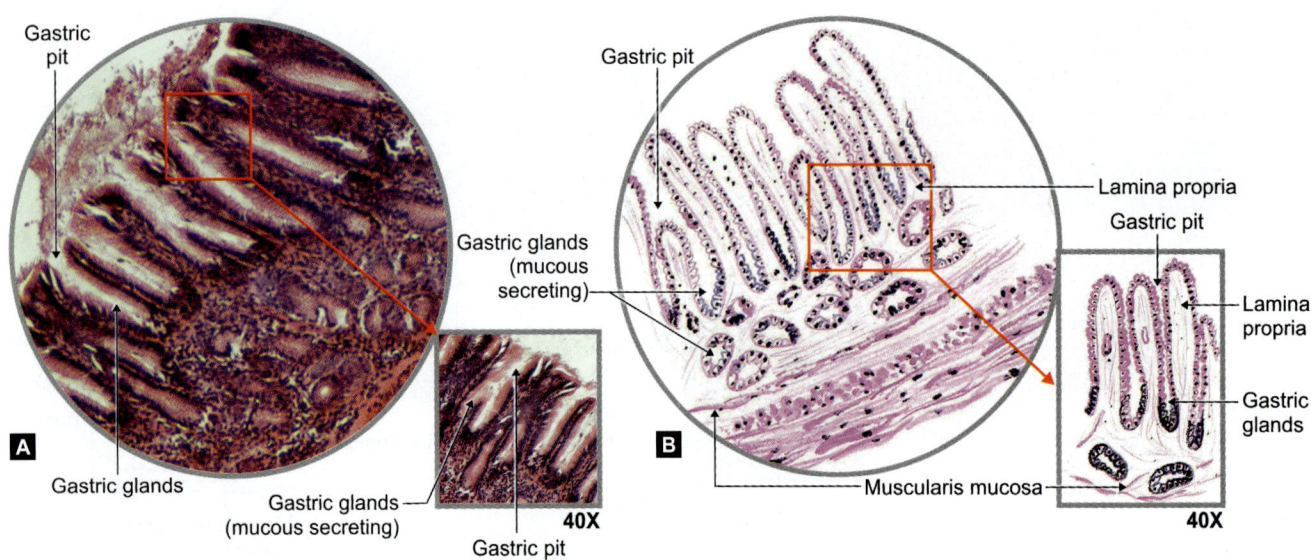

Figs 13.16A and B: (A) Microphotograph: Stomach (Pyloric)(20X); (B) Diagrammatic representation

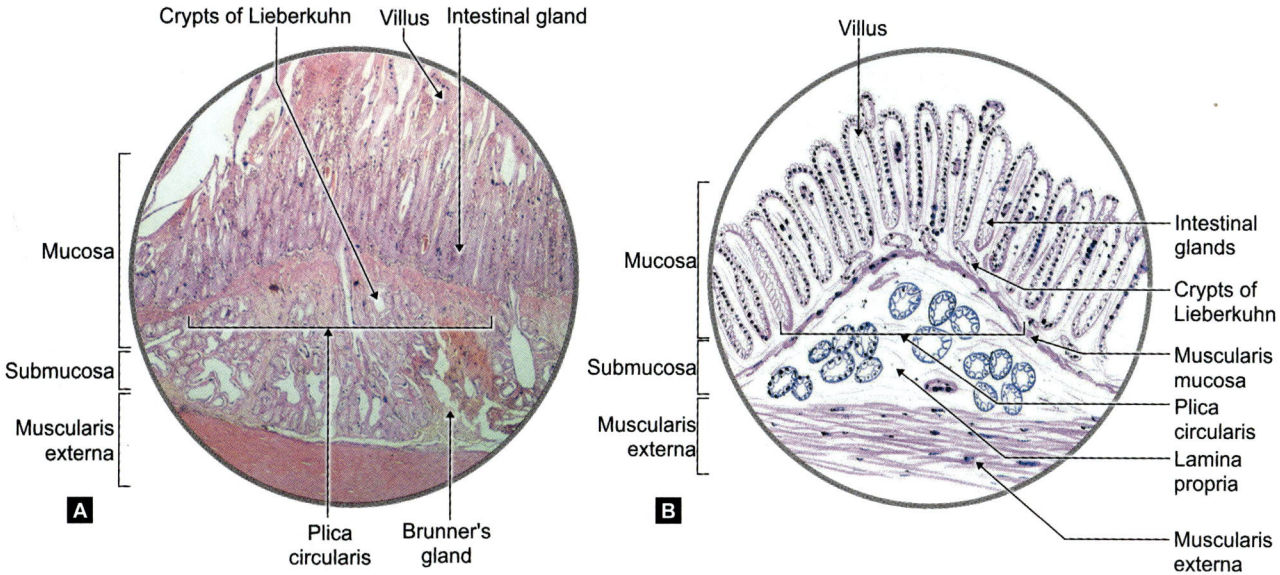

Figs 13.17A and B: (A) Microphotograph: Duodenum (4X); (B) Diagrammatic representation

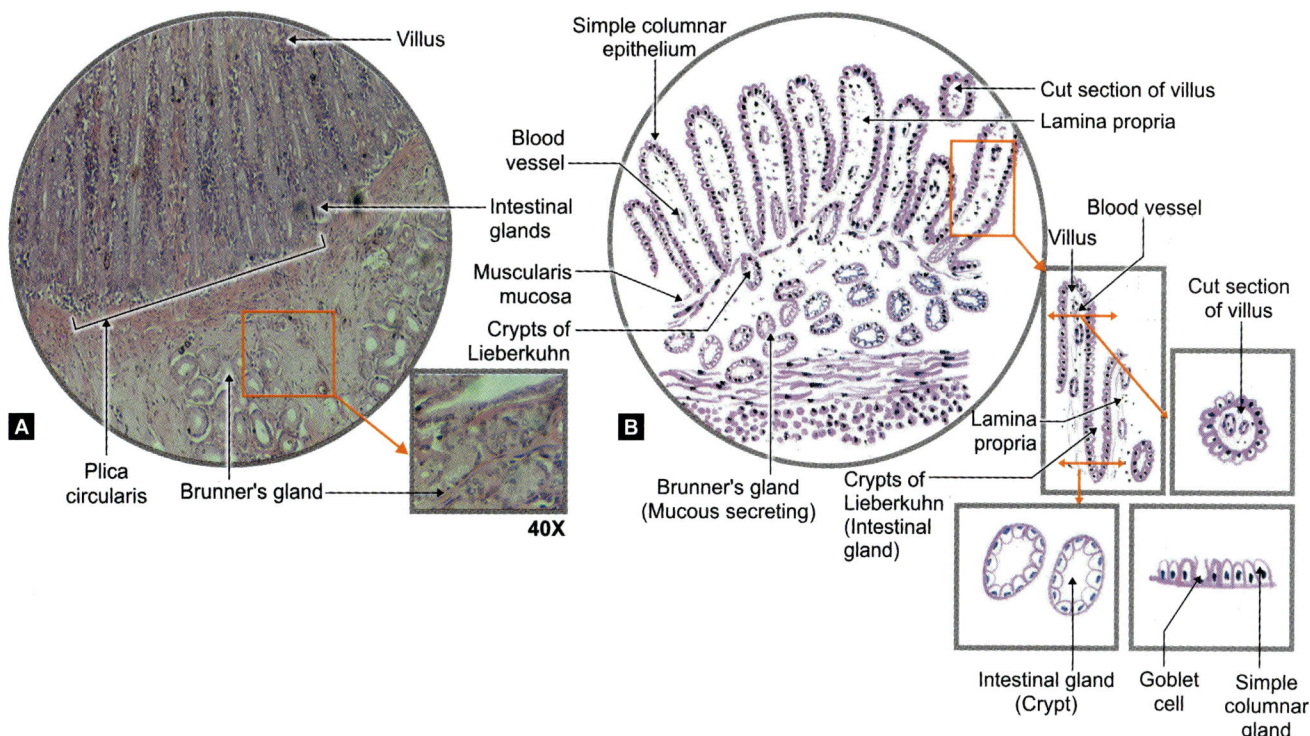

Figs 13.18A and B: (A) Microphotograph: Duodenum (20X); (B) Diagrammatic representation

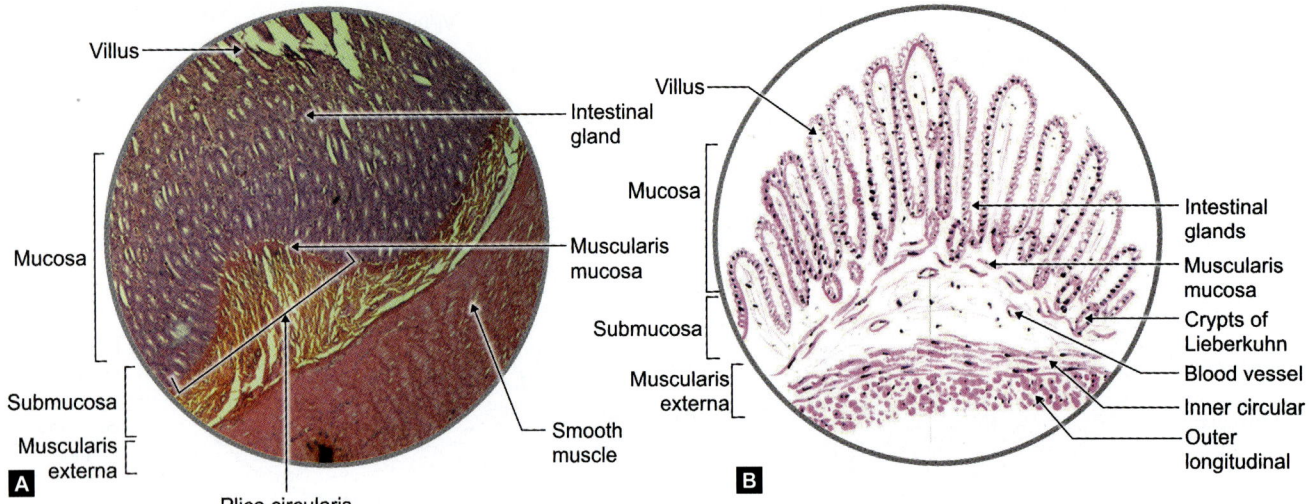

Figs 13.19A and B: (A) Microphotograph: Jejunum (4X); (B) Diagrammatic representation

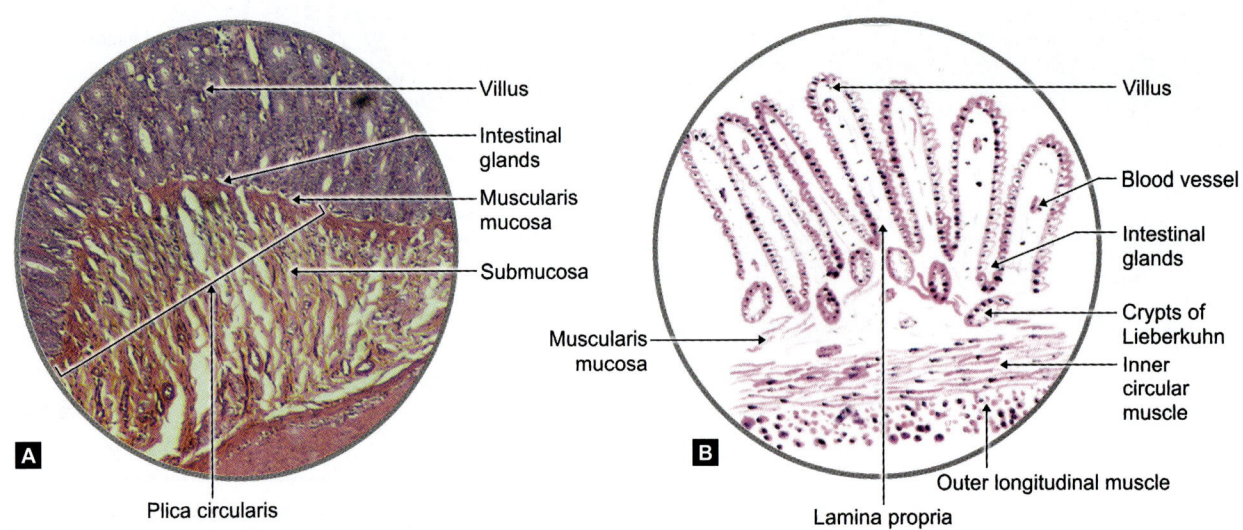

Figs 13.20A and B: (A) Microphotograph: Jejunum (20X); (B) Diagrammatic representation

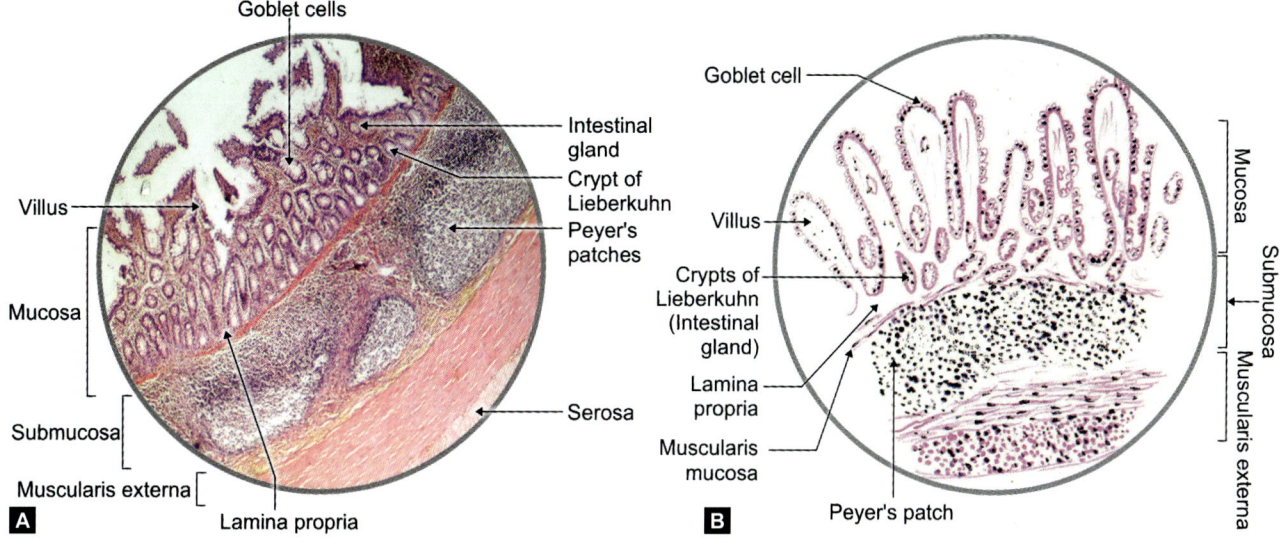

Figs 13.21A and B: (A) Microphotograph: Ileum (4X); (B) Diagrammatic representation

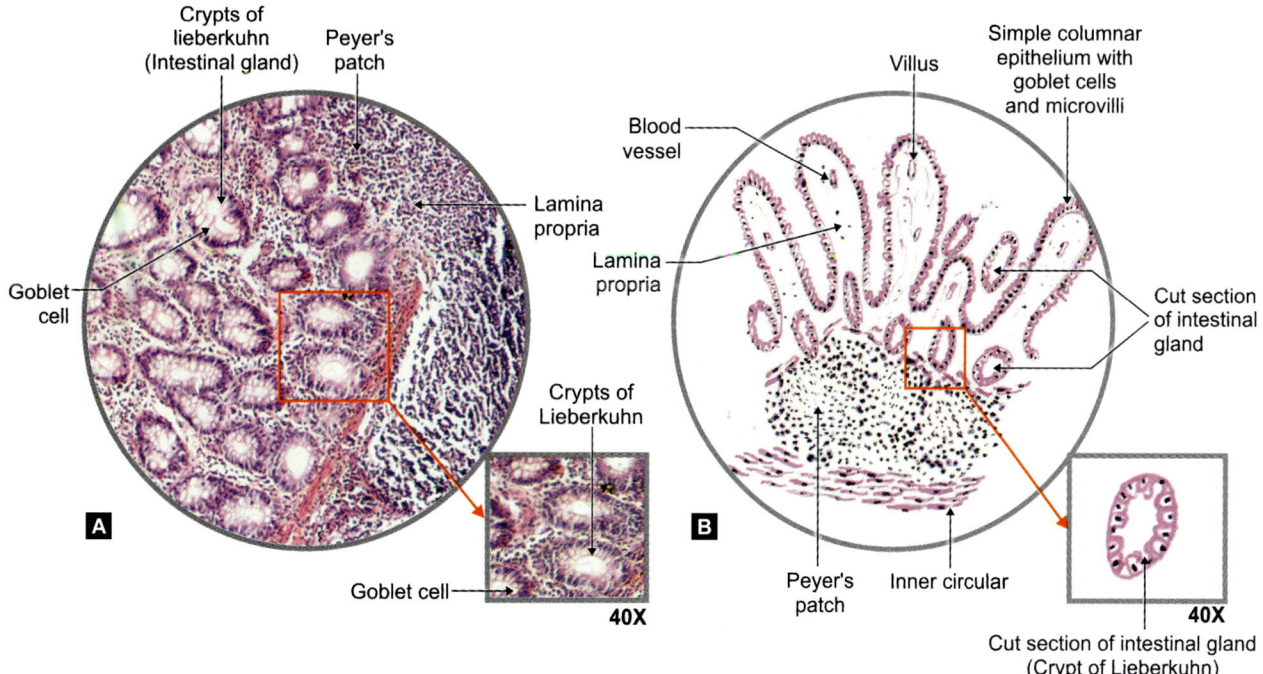

Figs 13.22A and B: (A) Microphotograph: Ileum (20X); (B) Diagrammatic representation

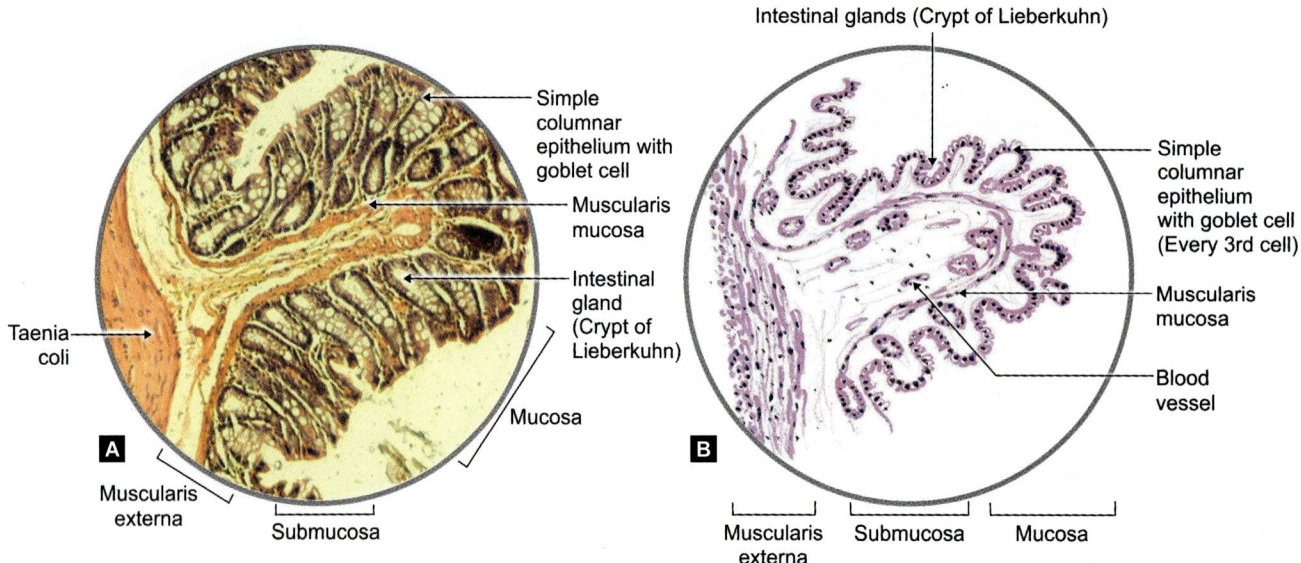

Figs 13.23A and B: (A) Microphotograph: Large intestine (4X); (B) Diagrammatic representation

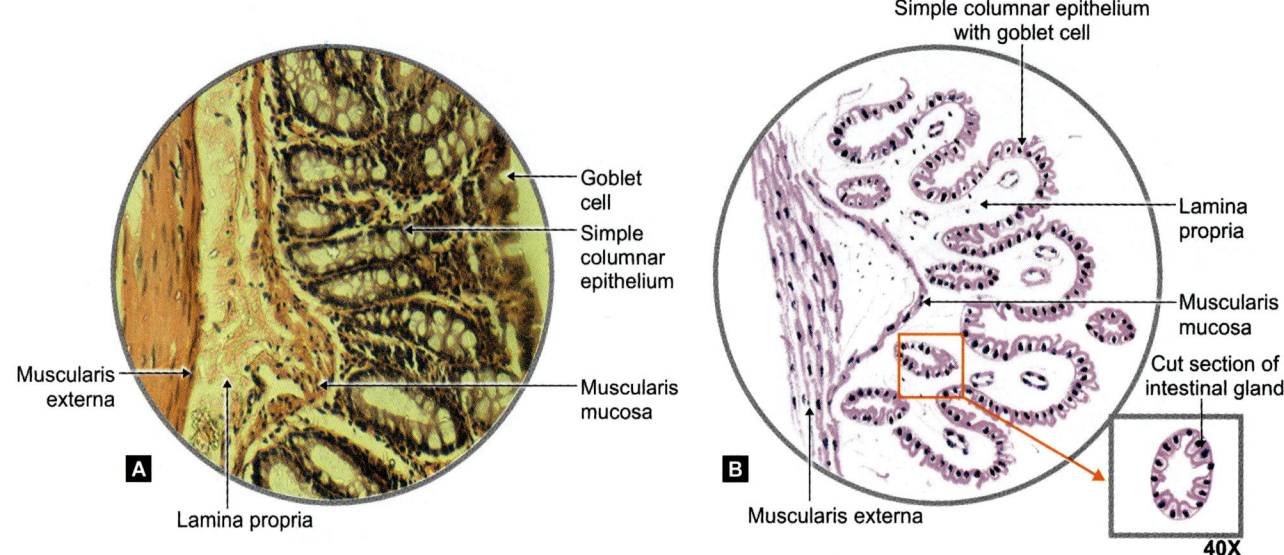

Figs 13.24A and B: (A) Microphotograph: Large intestine (20X); (B) Diagrammatic representation

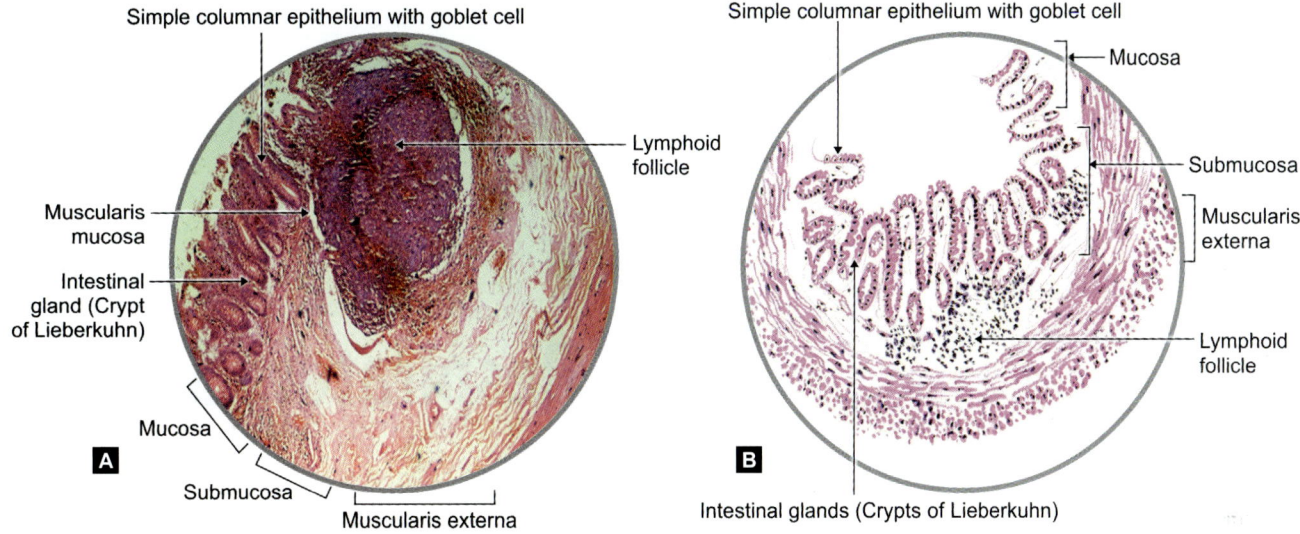

Figs 13.25A and B: (A) Microphotograph: Appendix (4X); (B) Diagrammatic representation

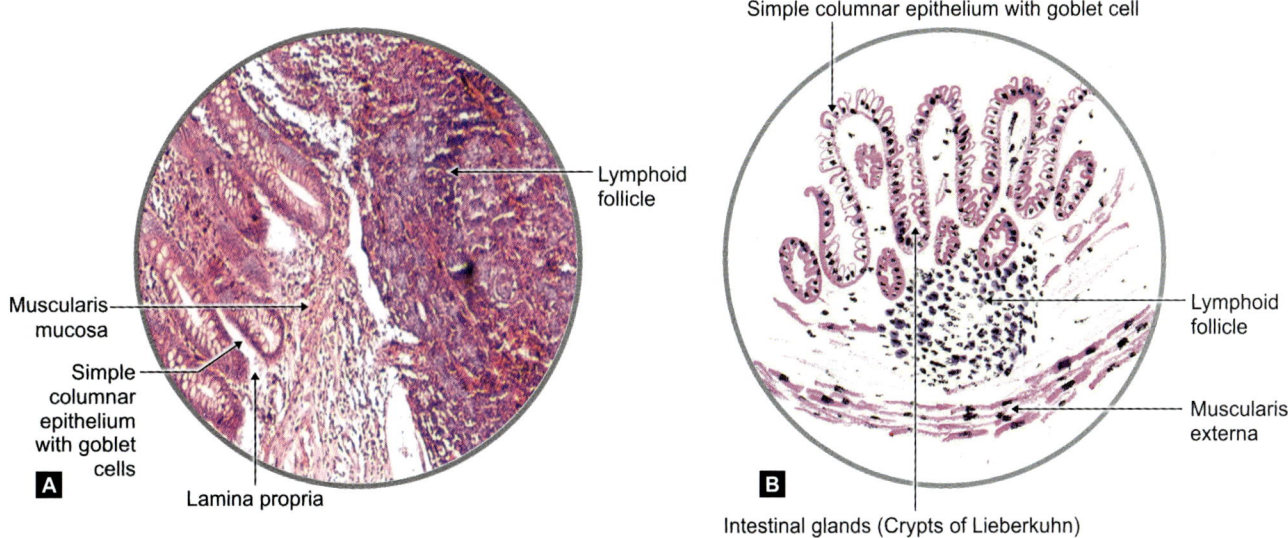

Figs 13.26A and B: (A) Microphotograph: Appendix (20X); (B) Diagrammatic representation

CHAPTER 14

Respiratory System

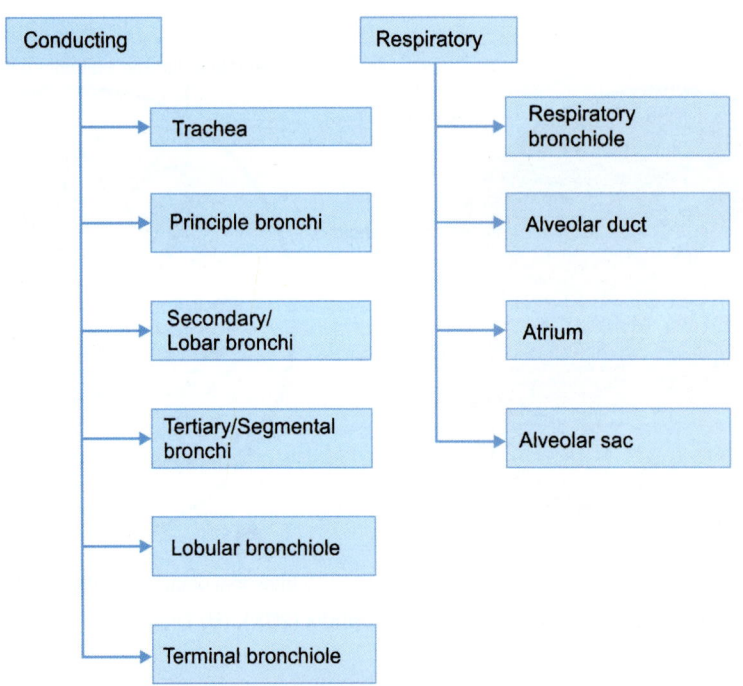

EPIGLOTTIS

- Elastic cartilage lined on either side by a mucous membrane *(Lip, tongue, eyelid are the other tissues lined by mucous membrane on either side but none of them show elastic cartilage inside)*
- Perichondrium of the elastic cartilage is continuous with the lamina propria on both the sides
- Anterior surface shows stratified squamous non-keratinised epithelium.

TABLE 14.1: Differentiating features of various parts of conducting respiratory system

	Extrapulmonary bronchus	Intrapulmonary bronchus	Bronchiole	Terminal bronchiole	Respiratory bronchiole	Alveoli
Epithelium	Pseudostratified ciliated	Pseudostratified ciliated	Ciliated columnar	Columnar with few cilia	Cuboidal cells (non-ciliated), Pouches of squamous cells	Simple squamous
Goblet cells	+	+	--	--	--	--
Clara cells	--	--	--	+	+	--
Submucosal glands	+	+	+	--	--	--
Smooth muscle	+	+	+	+	+ (not in alveolar sac)	--
Cartilage	+	+	--	--	--	--
Basal cells	+	+	--	--	--	--

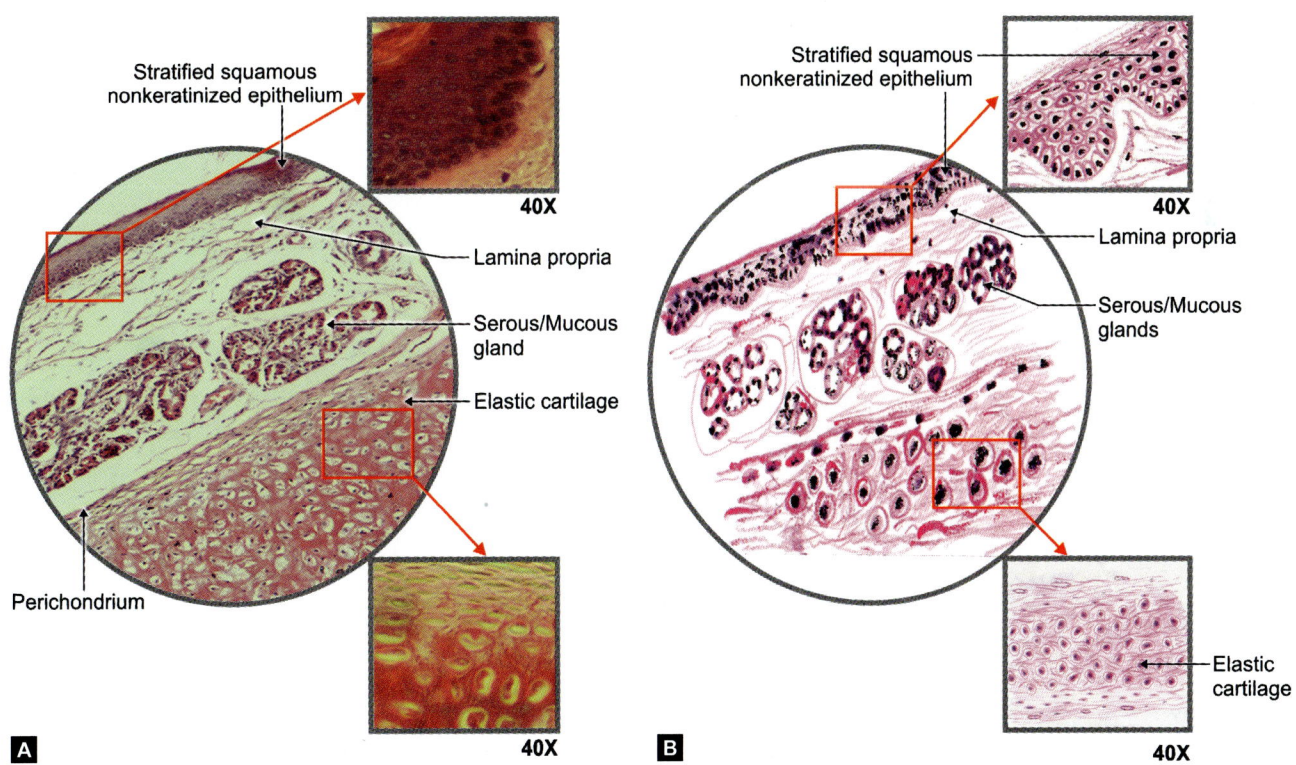

Figs 14.1A and B: (A) Microphotograph: Epiglottis (4X, 20X); (B) Diagrammatic representation

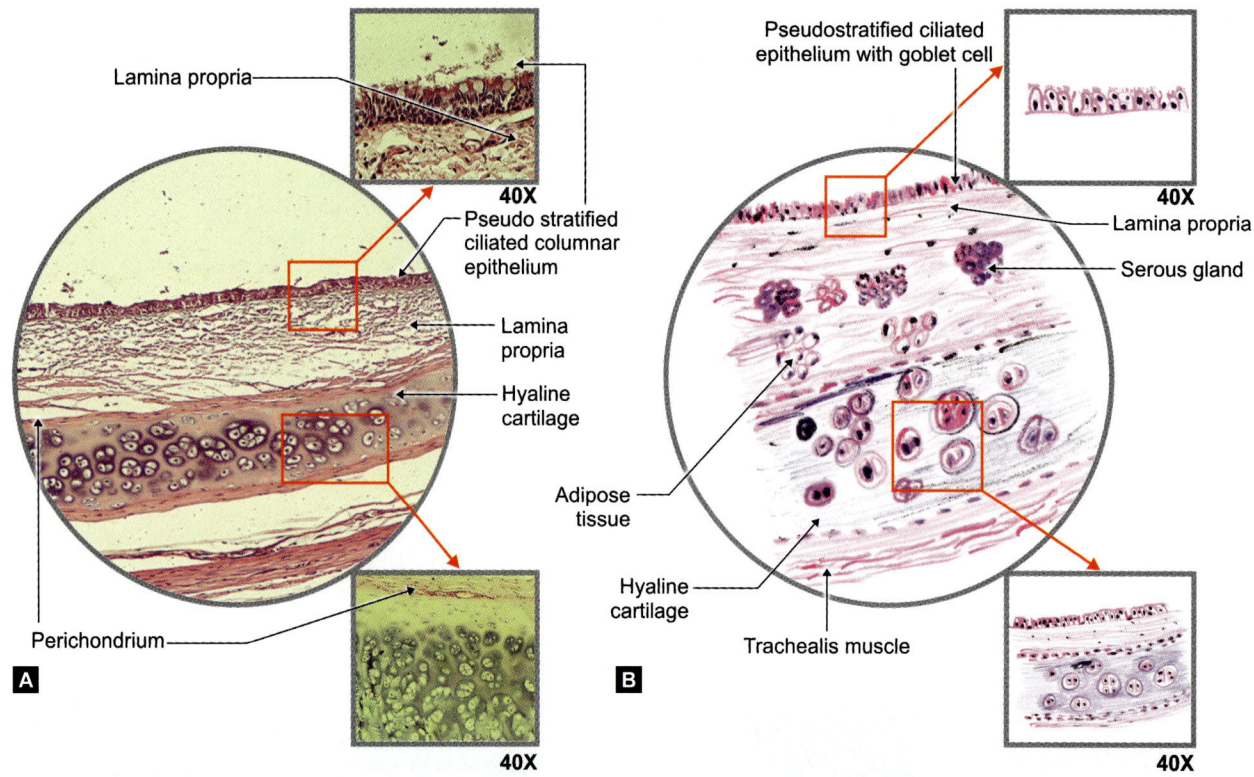

Figs 14.2A and B: (A) Microphotograph: Trachea (4X, 20X); (B) Diagrammatic representation

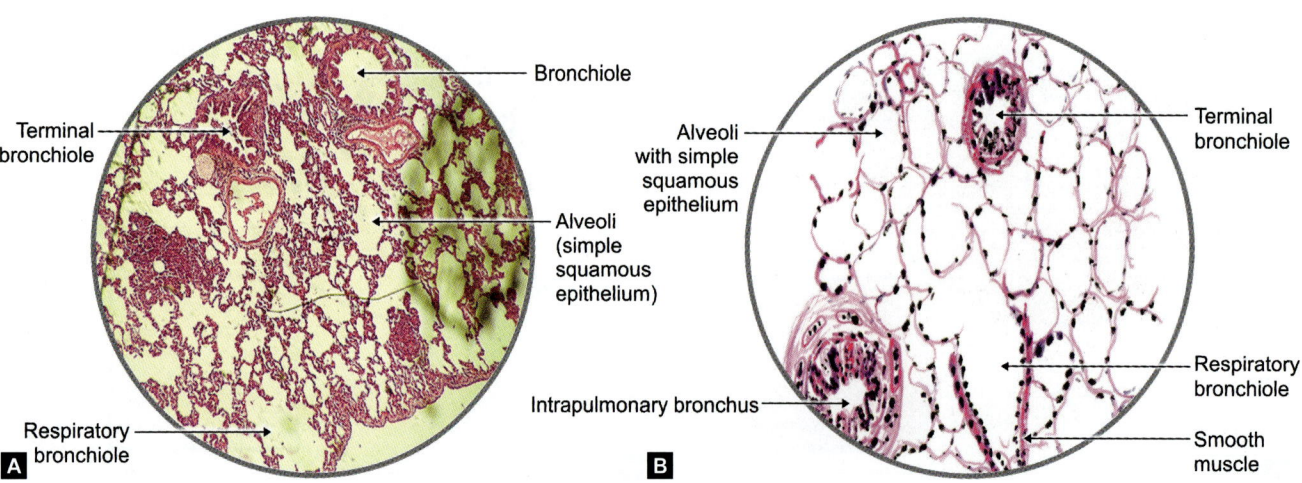

Figs 14.3A and B: (A) Microphotograph: Lung (4X); (B) Diagrammatic representation

Respiratory System

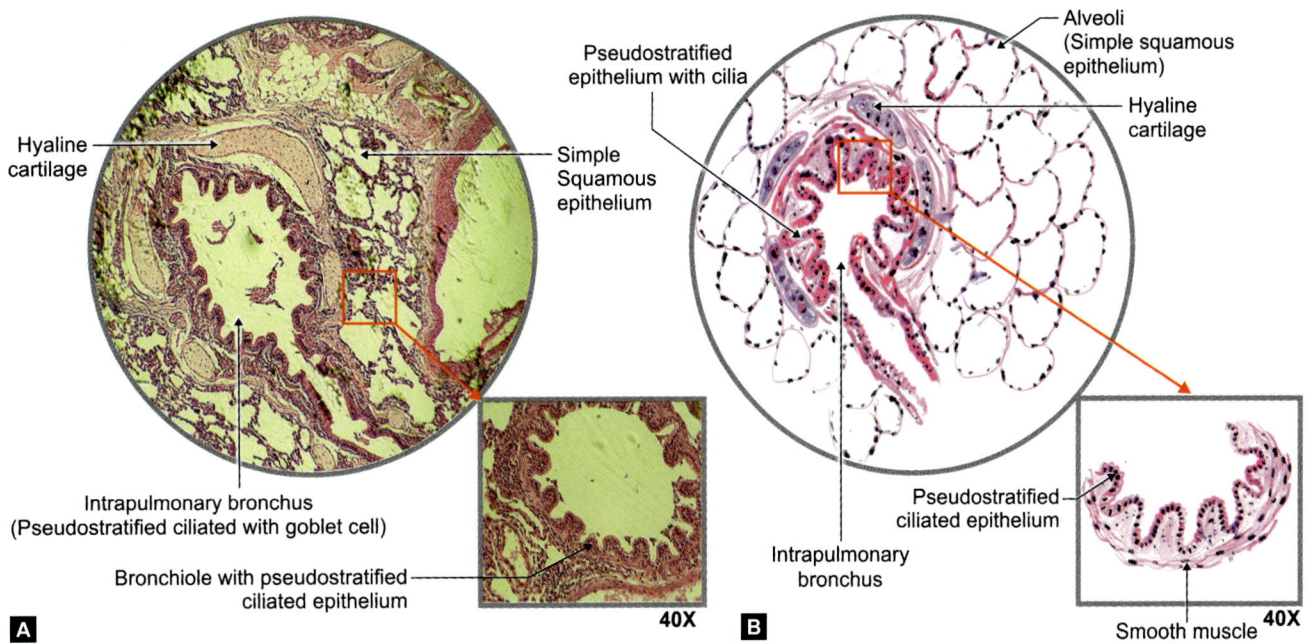

Figs 14.4A and B: (A) Microphotograph: Lung (20X); (B) Diagrammatic representation

CHAPTER 15

Urinary System

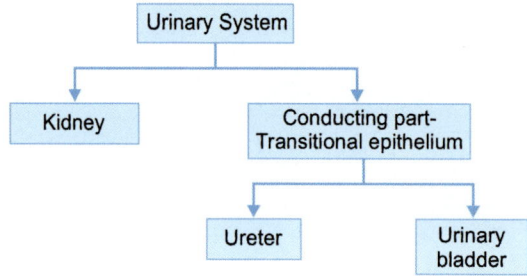

KIDNEY

Kidney is covered by fibrous capsule
Divided into outer cortex and inner medulla
Nephron shows:
- Cortex is pink, granular, darkly stained and contains
  - All glomeruli
    - A tuft of capillaries contained in Bowman's capsule
  - All proximal convoluted tubules (PCT)
    - Cells are large in size lined by simple columnar to cuboidal epithelium
    - Central prominent euchromatic nucleus
    - Dark (pink) eosinophilic cytoplasm
    - Show prominent brush border on the luminal side and vertical striations on the basal side
  - All distal convoluted tubules (DCT)
    - Prominent lumen lined by simple cuboidal epithelium (*no brush border*)
- Medulla is lightly stained and striated in appearance.
  - Shows loops of Henle (thin part: cuboidal cells, thick part: squamous)
  - Collecting tubules, all run fairly straight course (pale stained cuboidal cells)
  - Collecting ducts (columnar to cuboidal)

Nephron is the structural and functional unit of kidney.
- *Bowman's capsule with glomeruli, proximal and distal convoluted tubules and a loop of Henle*

  A conical pyramid of medullary substance together with the cap of cortical substance that covers its base constitutes a lobe of kidney.

URETER T.S.

Tubular structure with muscle wall *(can be easily distinguished from appendix, vas deferens, fallopian tubes, etc. by the presence of urothelium).*
Ureter wall shows three layers
- Innermost layer is mucous membrane:
  - Transitional epithelium and lamina propria *(epithelium has the ability to become thinner and flatter to accommodate for distension by urine)*
  - Mucous membrane is thrown into folds so that the lumen is star shaped in T.S.
- Smooth muscle layer:
  - Inner longitudinal
  - Outer circular
- Serosa/Adventitia.

URINARY BLADDER

It shows same three layers like that of the ureter.
- Innermost layer is mucous membrane:
  - The lumen lined by transitional epithelium (can be stretched without being damaged)
  - The stretched epithelium is thinner and the cells are flattened, while relaxed epithelium shows umbrella like cells
- Smooth muscle layer (Detrusor):
  - Inner longitudinal,
  - Outer circular and
  - Outermost longitudinal layer
- Serosa/Adventitia.

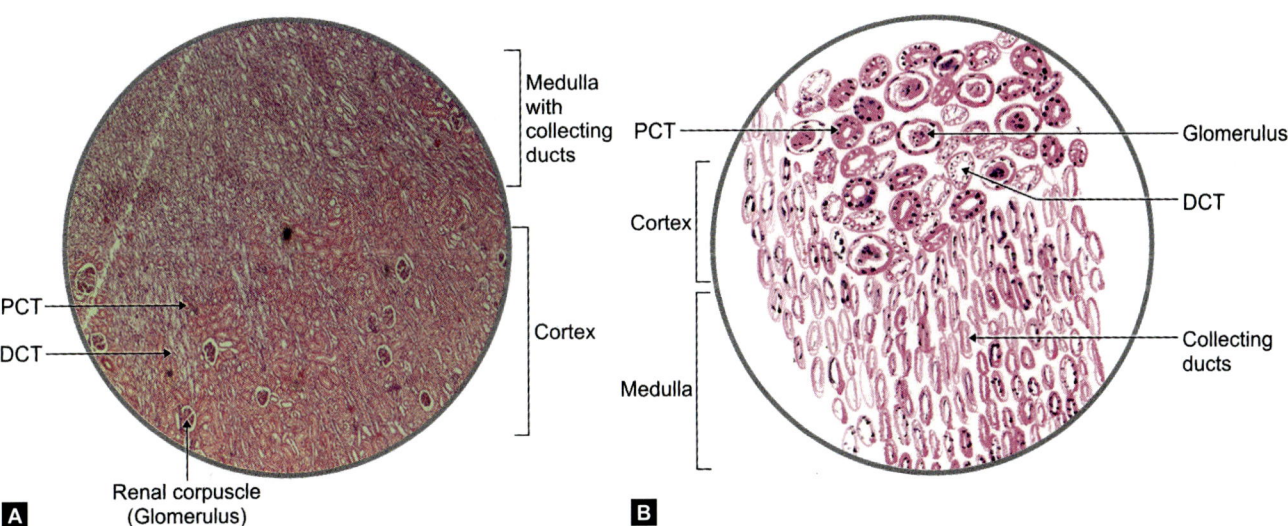

Figs 15.1A and B: (A) Microphotograph: Kidney (4X); (B) Diagrammatic representation

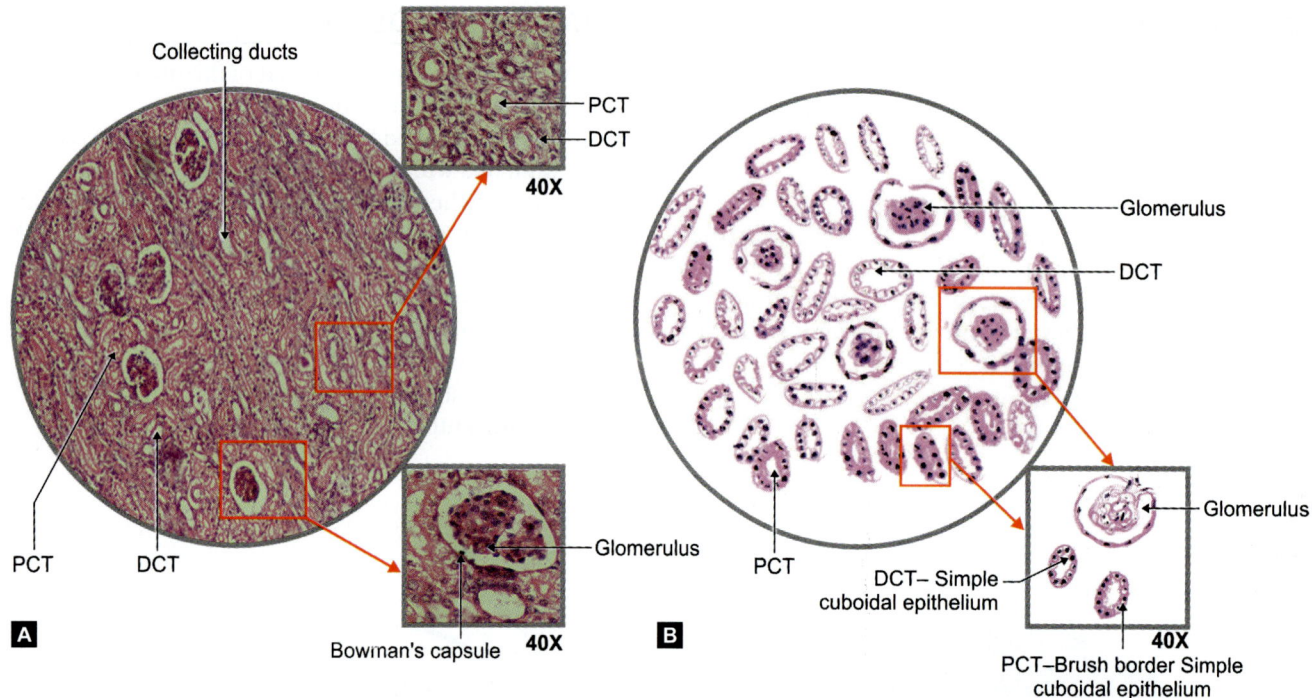

Figs 15.2A and B: (A) Microphotograph: Kidney (20X); (B) Diagrammatic representation

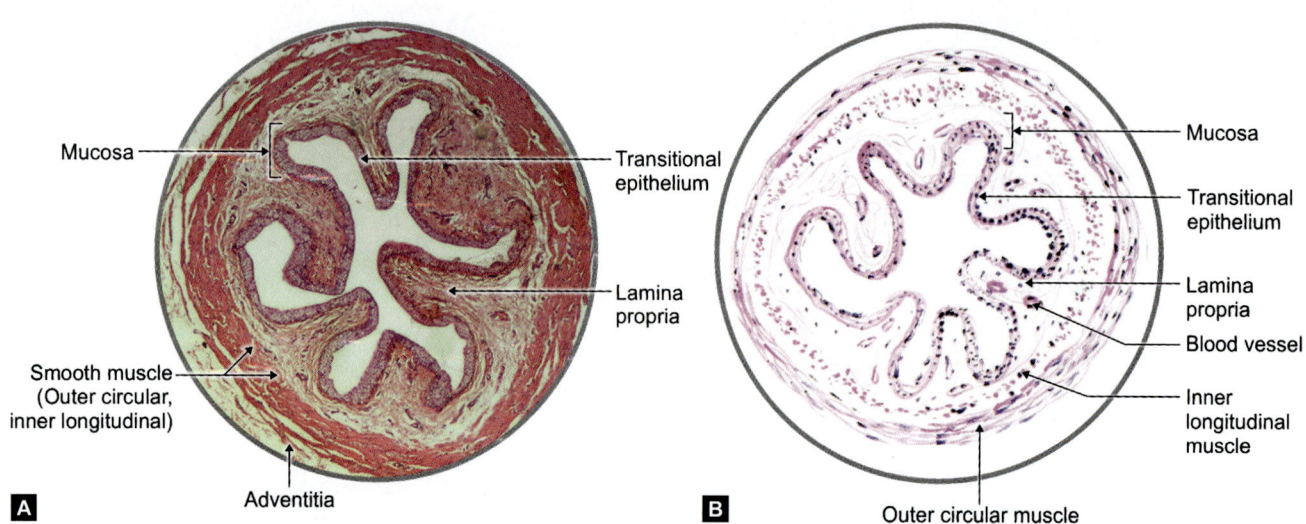

Figs 15.3A and B: (A) Microphotograph: Ureter (4X); (B) Diagrammatic representation

Urinary System

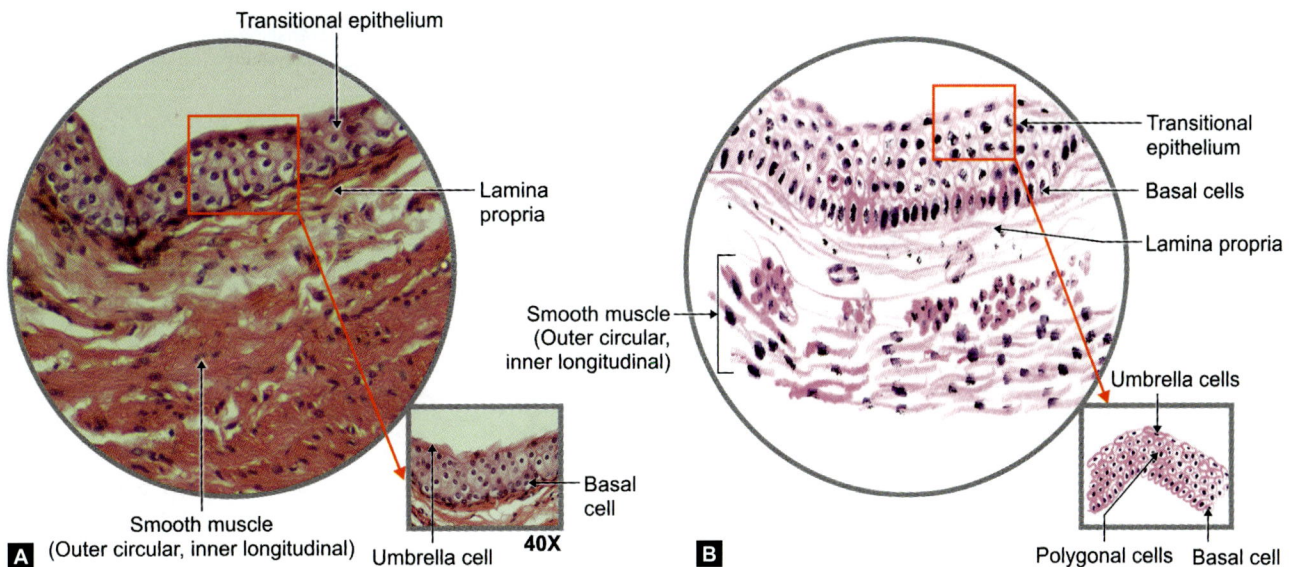

Figs 15.4A and B: (A) Microphotograph: Ureter (20X); (B) Diagrammatic representation

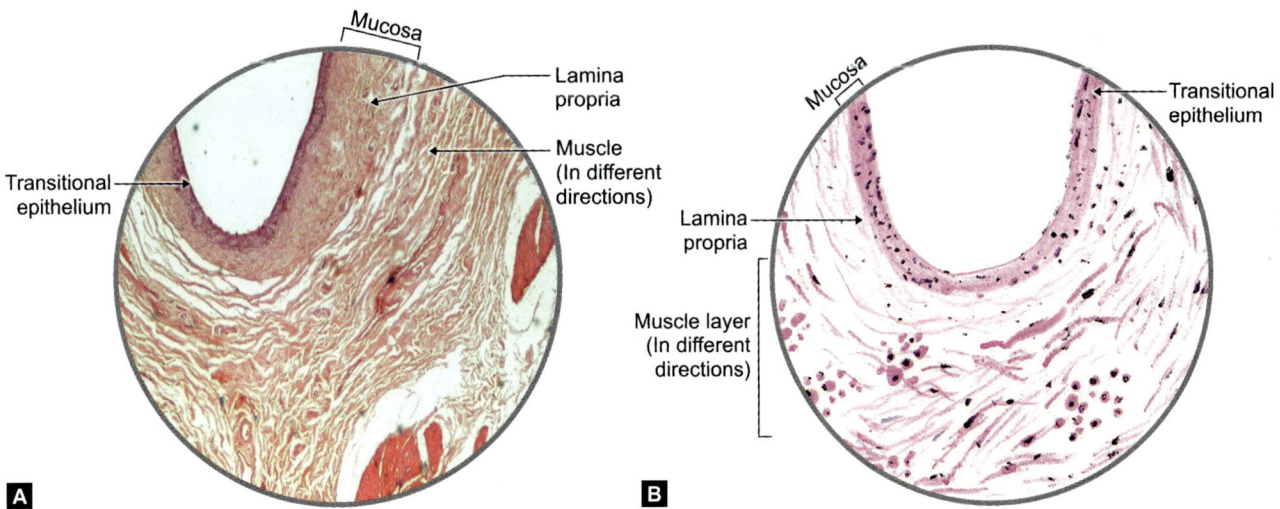

Figs 15.5A and B: (A) Microphotograph: Urinary bladder (4X); (B) Diagrammatic representation

68 Atlas of Histology for Medical Students

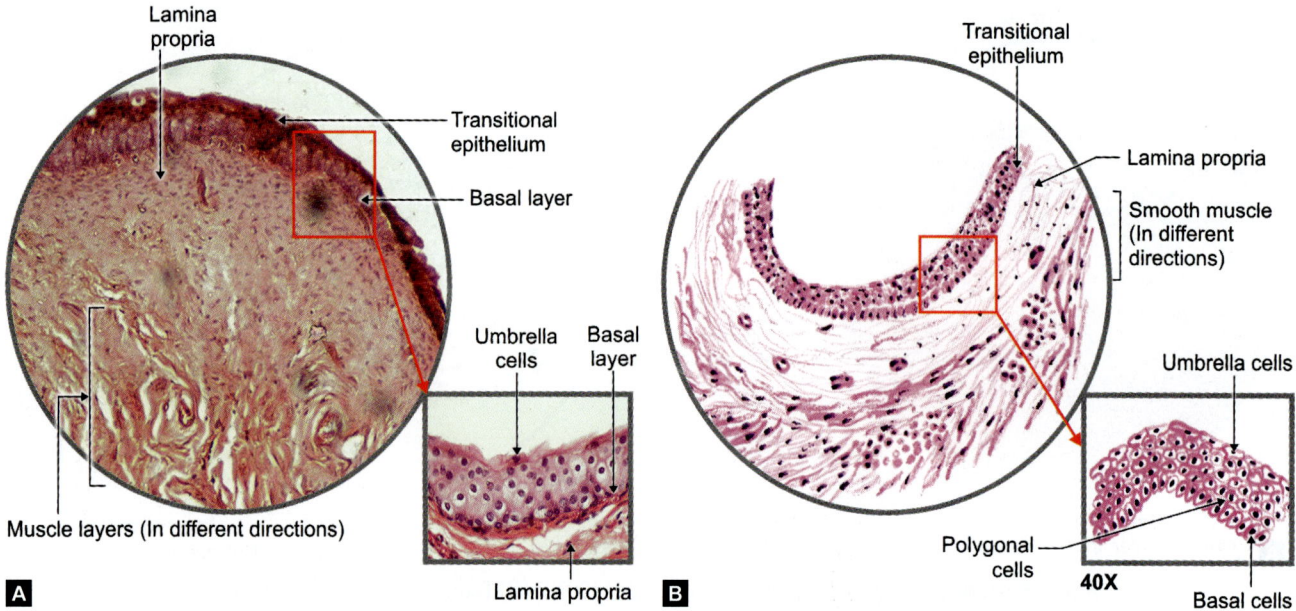

Figs 15.6A and B: (A) Microphotograph: Urinary bladder (20X); (B) Diagrammatic representation

CHAPTER 16

Male Reproductive System

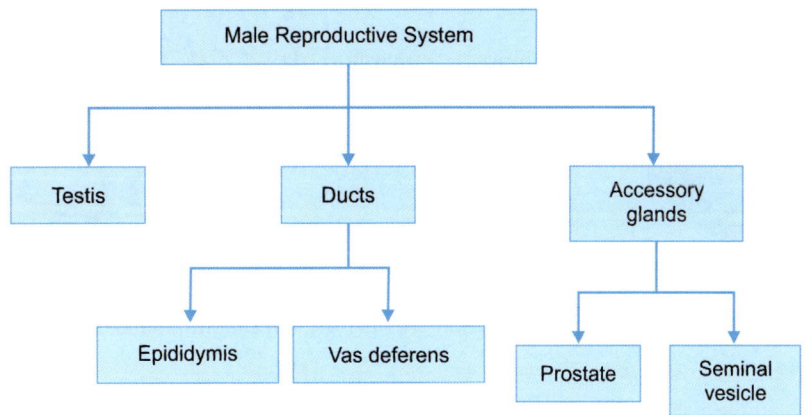

TESTIS

- Testis is enclosed in a thick connective tissue capsule (Tunica albuginea)
- Fibrous septa divide the tissue into lobules containing seminiferous tubules
- Seminiferous tubules
  - Long convoluted lined by germinal epithelium
  - Contain two types of cells:
    - Spermatogenic cells in various stages, sperms
    - Supportive cells (Sertoli cells) that nourish the developing sperm
- Interstitial cells of Leydig
  - Located in the connective tissue
  - Secrete testosterone.

DUCTUS DEFERENS

Ductus deferens exhibits narrow and irregular lumen with longitudinal folds
- Mucosa
  - Pseudostratified columnar epithelium with stereocilia
- Muscular coat consists of 3 layers:
  - Inner longitudinal
  - Middle circular
  - Outer longitudinal
- Adventitia- Outermost layer.

EPIDIDYMIS

- Long convoluted tubules
  - Pseudostratified columnar epithelium (tall columnar cells with stereocilia, small basal cells)
- Tubules of epididymis are surrounded by a thin layer of smooth muscle fibers.

PROSTATE

It is a fibromusculoglandular tissue
- Glands
  - Glandular acini (simple columnar, light stained)
  - Lumen wide and generally irregular *(contain spherical concretions called corpora amylacea or amyloid bodies)*
  - Excretory ducts resemble acini with simple columnar epithelium but cells stain darker
- Fibromuscular stroma.

SEMINAL VESICLE

Highly convoluted and irregular lumen
- Mucosa
  - Primary and secondary mucosal folds
  - Epithelium is low pseudo stratified to low columnar or cuboidal
- Muscular layer
  - Inner circular
  - Outer longitudinal.

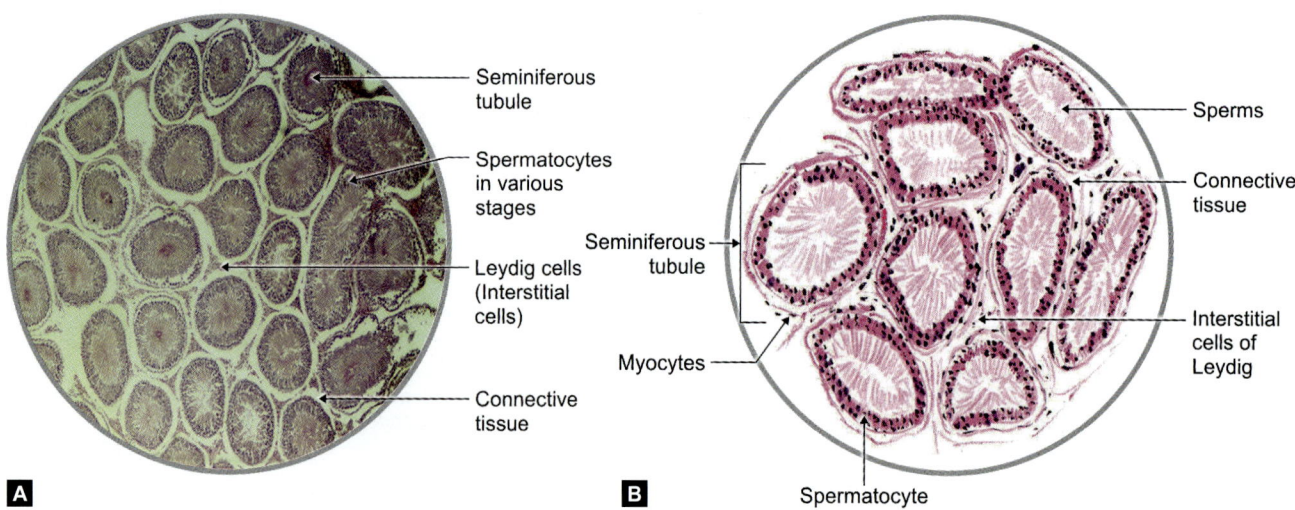

Figs 16.1A and B: (A) Microphotograph: Testis (4X); (B) Diagrammatic representation

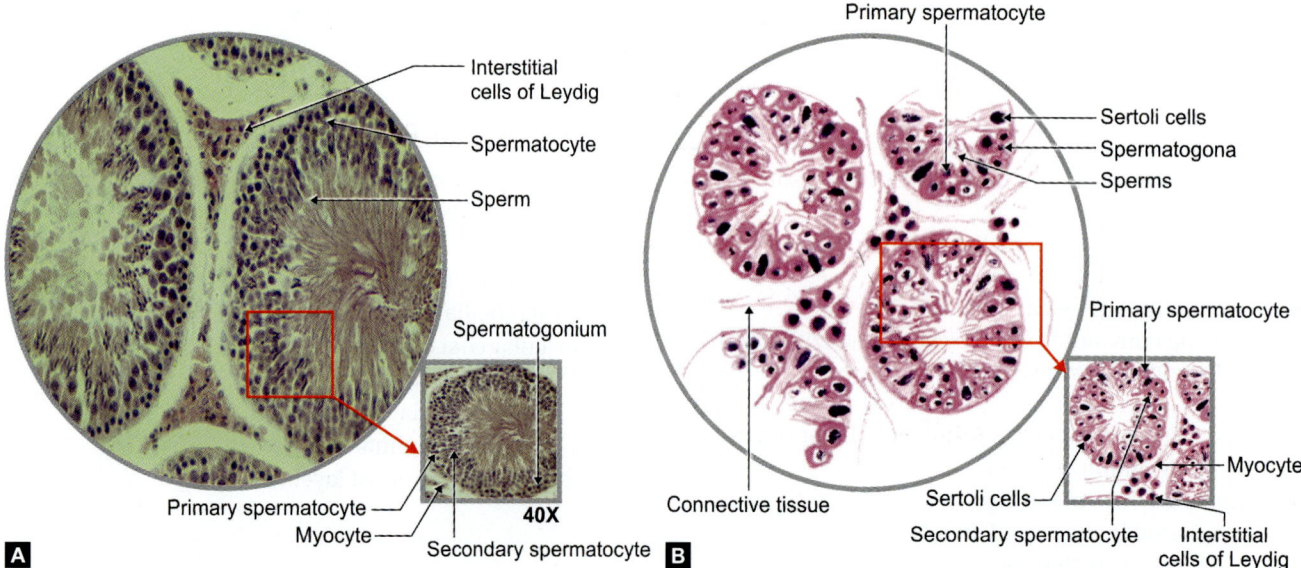

Figs 16.2A and B: (A) Microphotograph: Testis (20X); (B) Diagrammatic representation

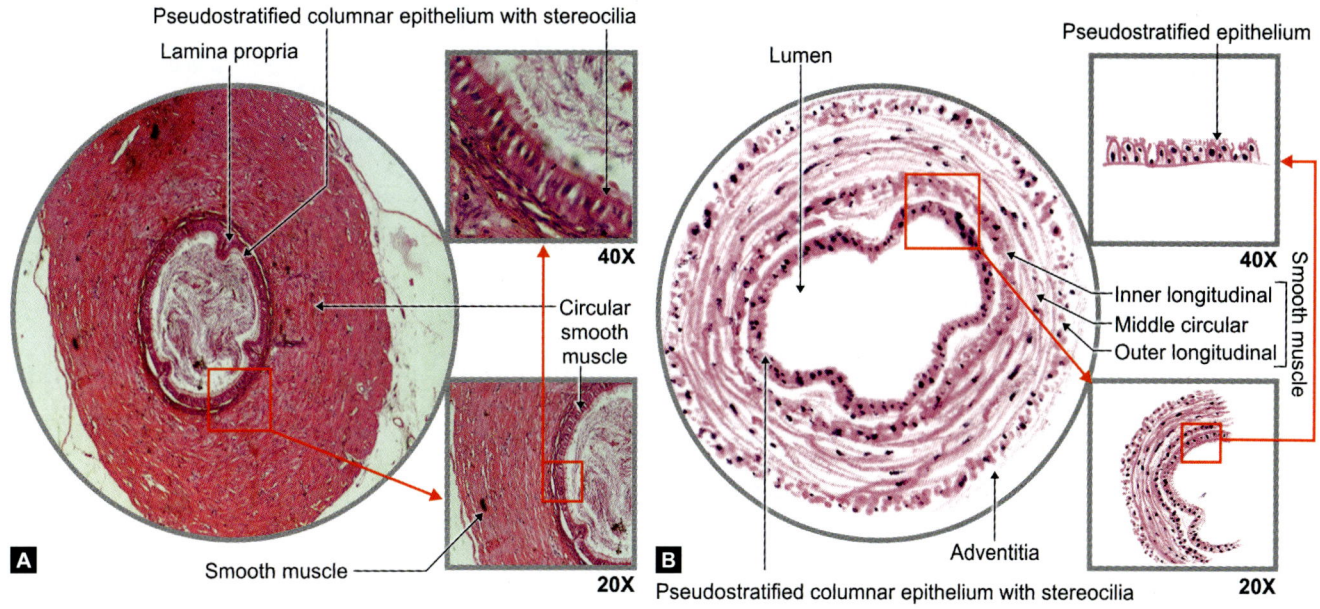

Figs 16.3A and B: (A) Microphotograph: Ductus deferens (4X, 20X); (B) Diagrammatic representation

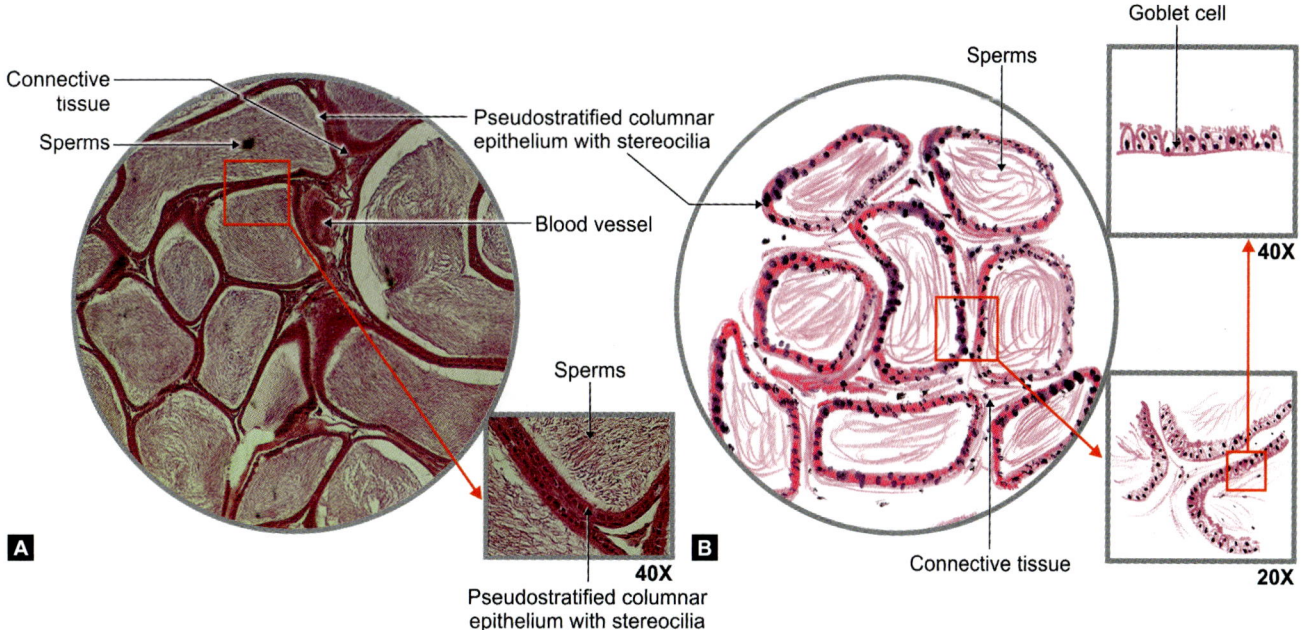

Figs 16.4A and B: (A) Microphotograph: Epididymis (4X, 20X); (B) Diagrammatic representation

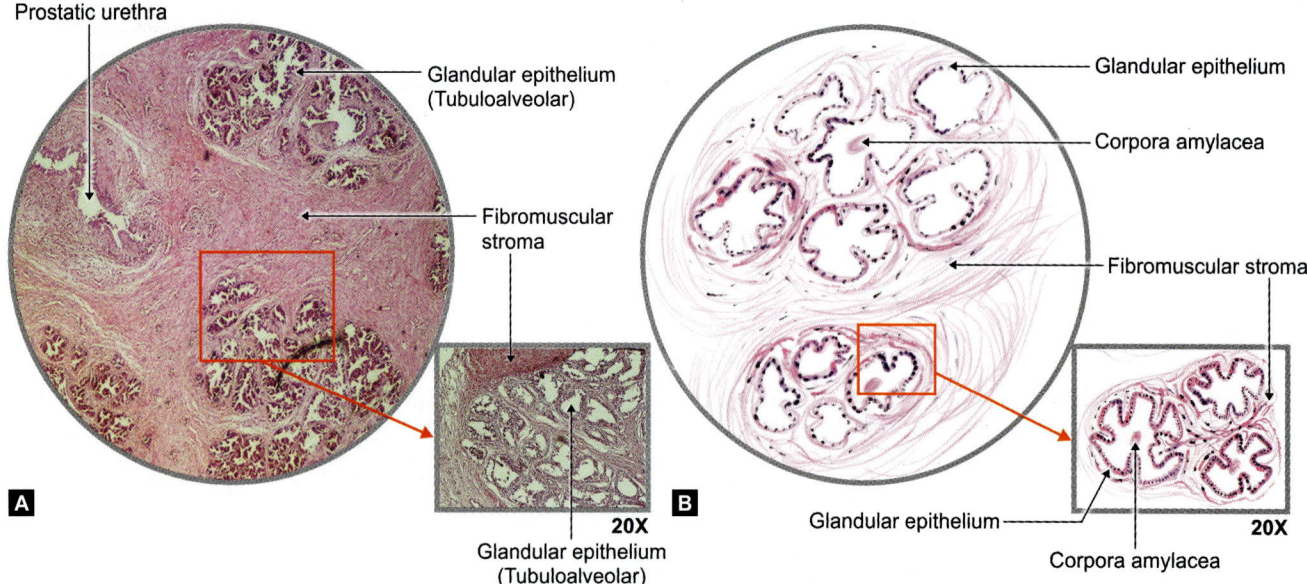

Figs 16.5A and B: (A) Microphotograph: Prostate (4X, 20X); (B) Diagrammatic representation

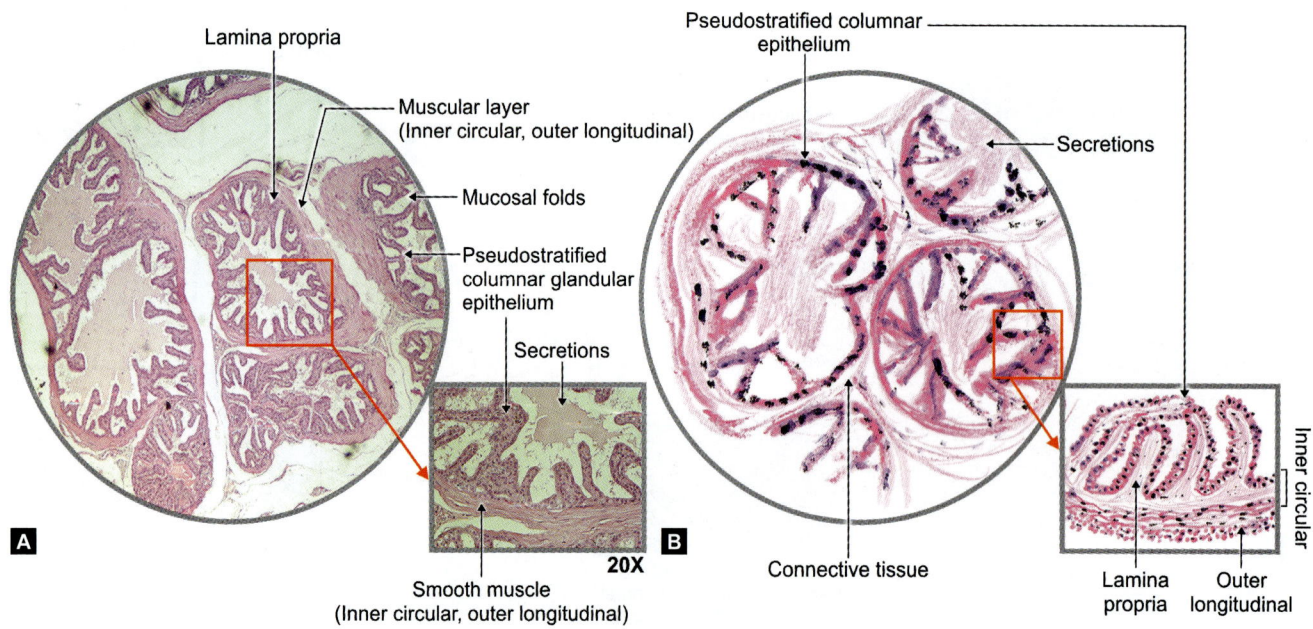

Figs 16.6A and B: (A) Microphotograph: Seminal vesicle (4X, 20X); (B) Diagrammatic representation

17 CHAPTER

Female Reproductive System

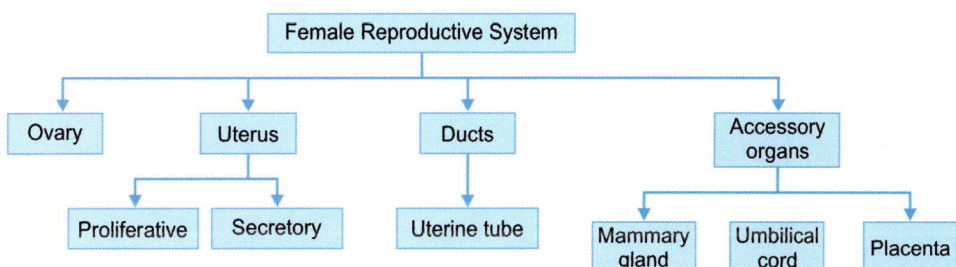

OVARY

Ovarian surface is covered by single layer of low cuboidal germinal epithelium (misnomer—It does not form germinal cells)
Divided into peripheral cortex and central medulla.
- Cortex:
  - Numerous ovarian follicles at various stages of development namely primordial (most numerous), primary, secondary and mature follicles.

  The largest follicle is the mature follicle which consists of theca interna, theca externa, granulosa cells, a large antrum with follicular fluid, and the cumulus oophorus that contains the primary oocyte
- Medulla:
  - In the center of the ovary
  - Contains loose connective tissue and blood vessels.

UTERUS

Uterus consists of three layers.
- Inner endometrium
  - Lined by simple columnar epithelium
  - Lamina propria is thick with simple tubular glands and stroma.

  The endometrium is divided into 2 layers- stratum functionalis and basalis.
  - In proliferative phase
    - Glands are straight and arteries less coiled
  - In secretory phase
    - Glands become convoluted and arteries highly coiled.
- Middle layer of smooth muscle (myometrium).
  - Thick layer of smooth muscle.
- Outer serous layer (perimetrium).

UTERINE TUBE

Extensive mucous folds form an irregular lumen in the uterine tube.
- Epithelium:
  - Simple columnar (ciliated and nonciliated)
- Muscular Layer:
  - Inner circular
  - Outer longitudinal
- Serosa:
  - Outermost layer.

MAMMARY GLAND

- Compound tubuloalveolar gland consisting many lobes
- Shows many alveoli - lined by simple cuboidal epithelium
- Intra and interlobular ducts
- Adipose tissue present.

PLACENTA

Shows cross section of villi.
- Villus consists of
  - Thin syncytiotrophoblastic cells and also cytotrophoblast
  - Basement membrane of foetal capillary
  - Endothelial cells of fetal capillary.

UMBILICAL CORD

Umbilical cord consists of mxymatous connective tissue Surrounding two umbilical arteries, 1 umbilical vein.

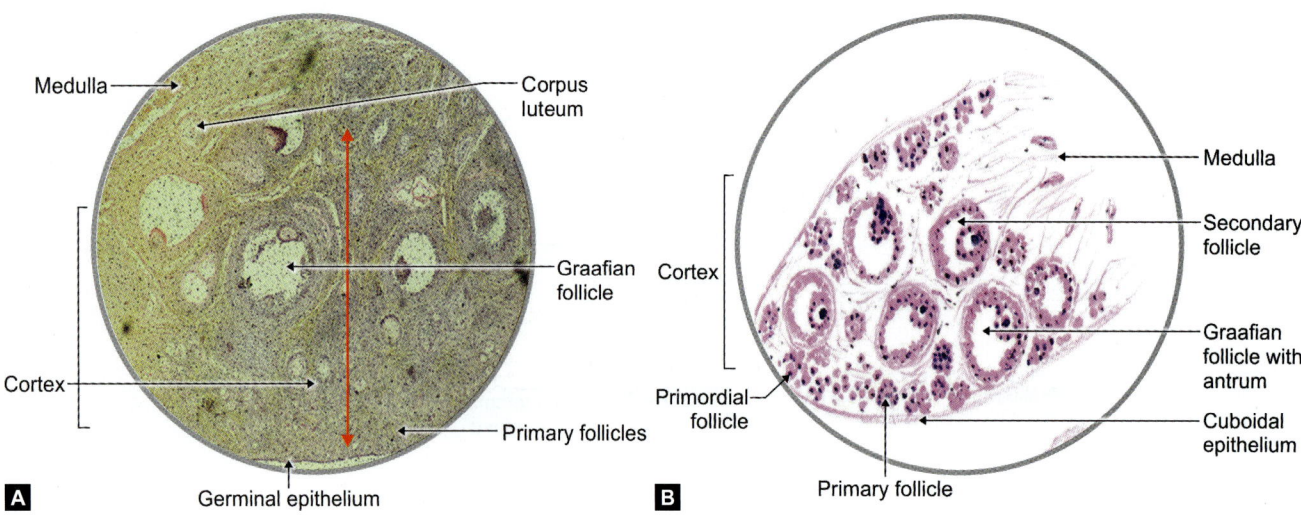

Figs 17.1A and B: (A) Microphotograph: Ovary (4X); (B) Diagrammatic representation

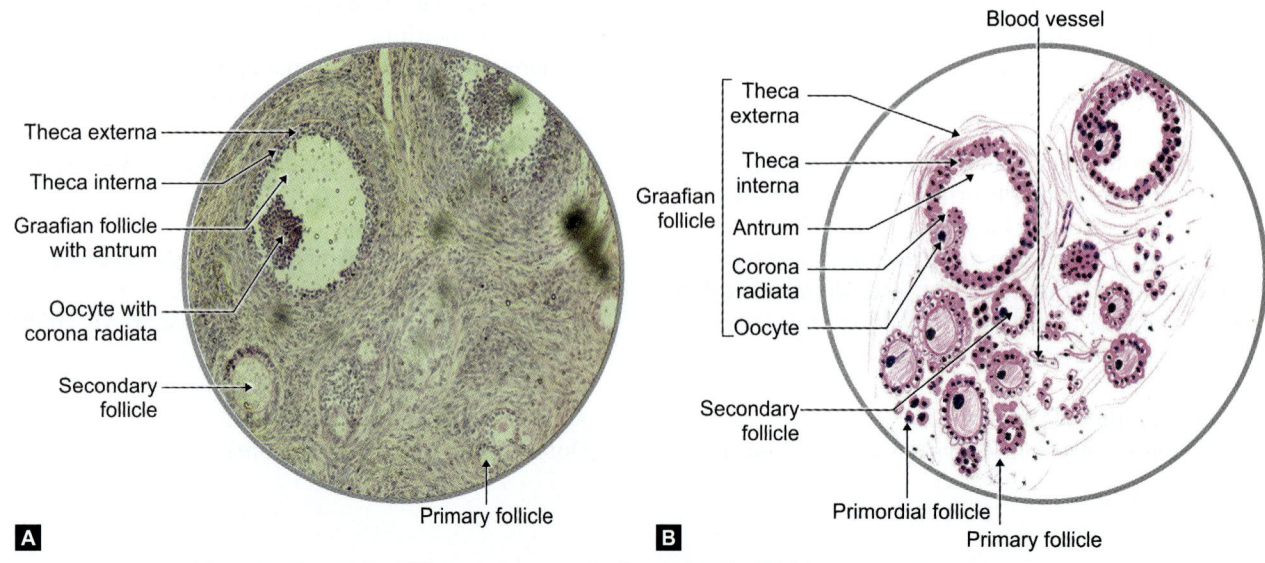

Figs 17.2A and B: (A) Microphotograph: Ovary (20X); (B) Diagrammatic representation

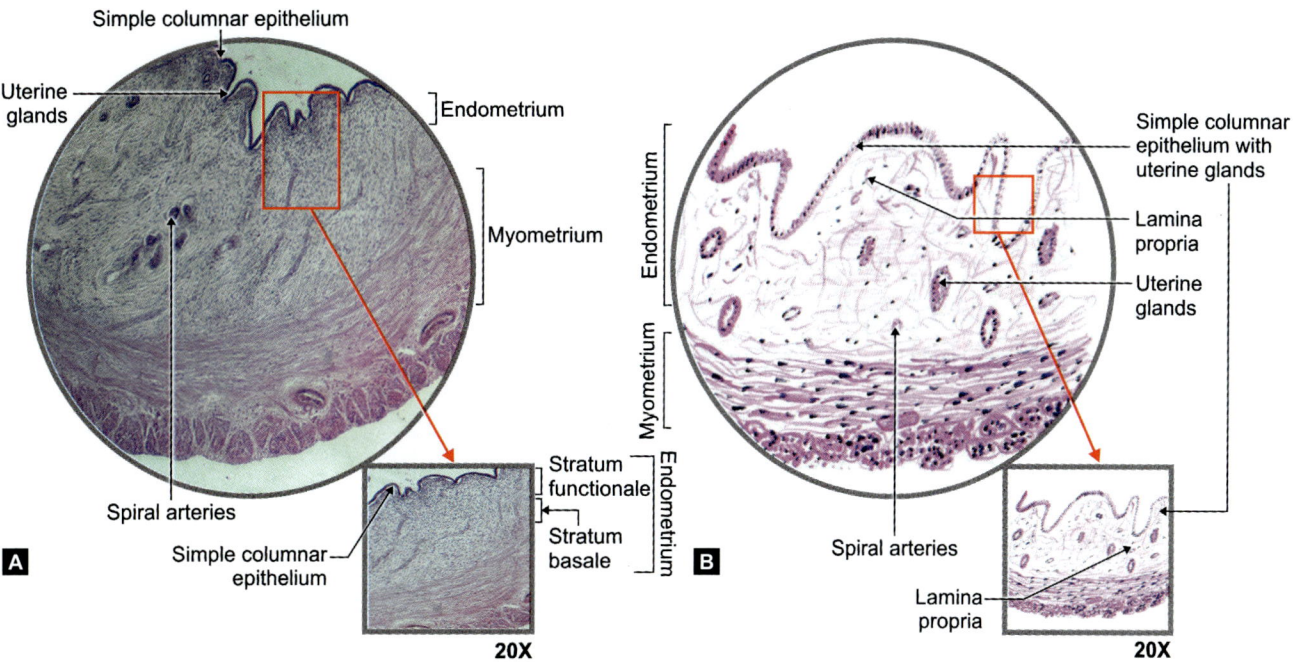

Figs 17.3A and B: (A) Microphotograph: Uterus (Proliferative phase)(4X, 20X); (B) Diagrammatic representation

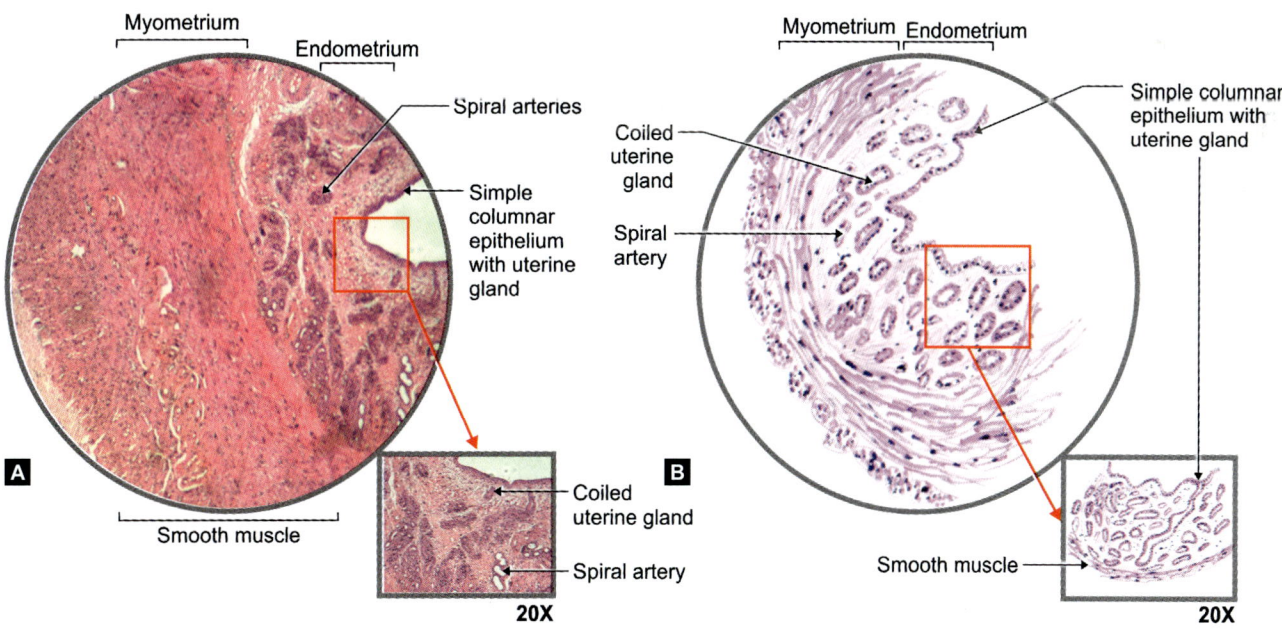

Figs 17.4A and B: (A) Microphotograph: Uterus (Secretory phase)(4X, 20X); (B) Diagrammatic representation

76 Atlas of Histology for Medical Students

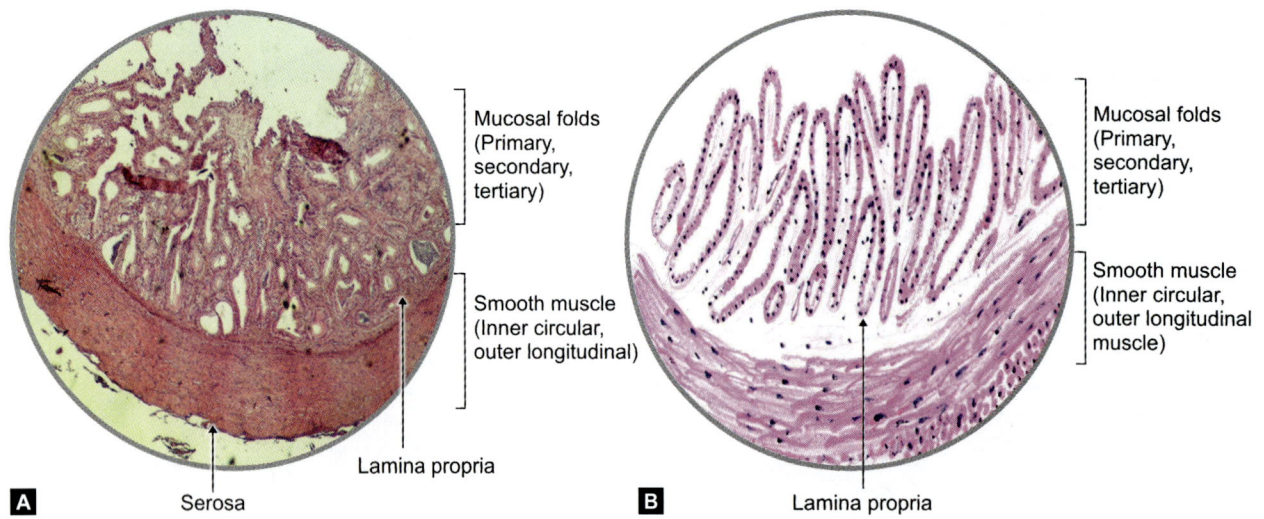

Figs 17.5A and B: (A) Microphotograph: Uterine tube (4X); (B) Diagrammatic representation

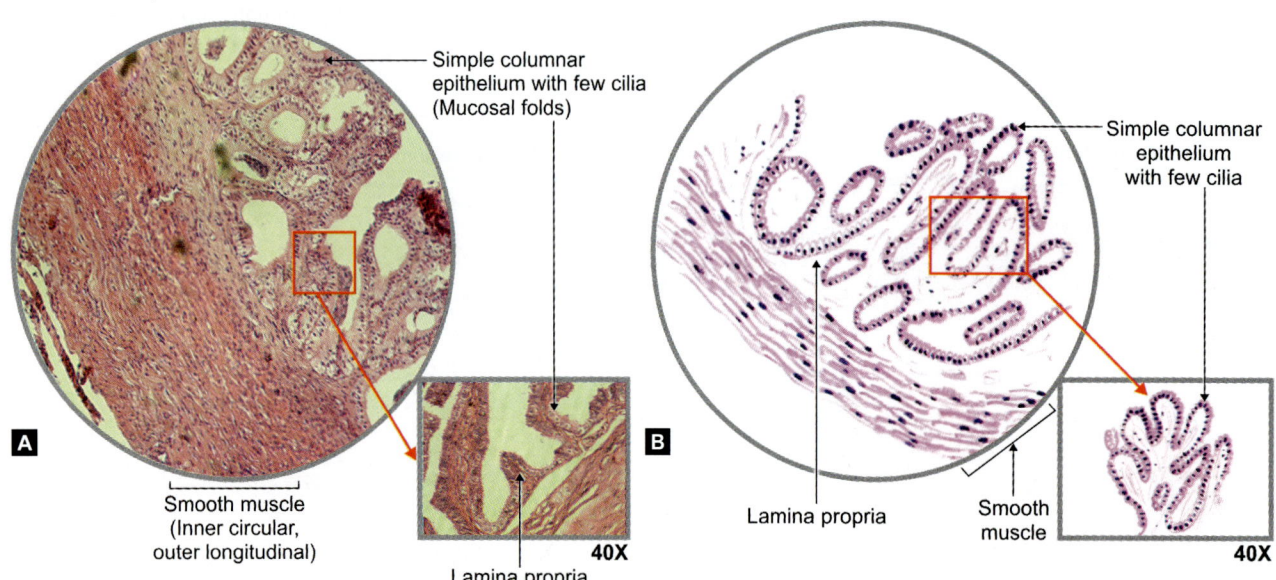

Figs 17.6A and B: (A) Microphotograph: Uterine tube (20X); (B) Diagrammatic representation

Female Reproductive System **77**

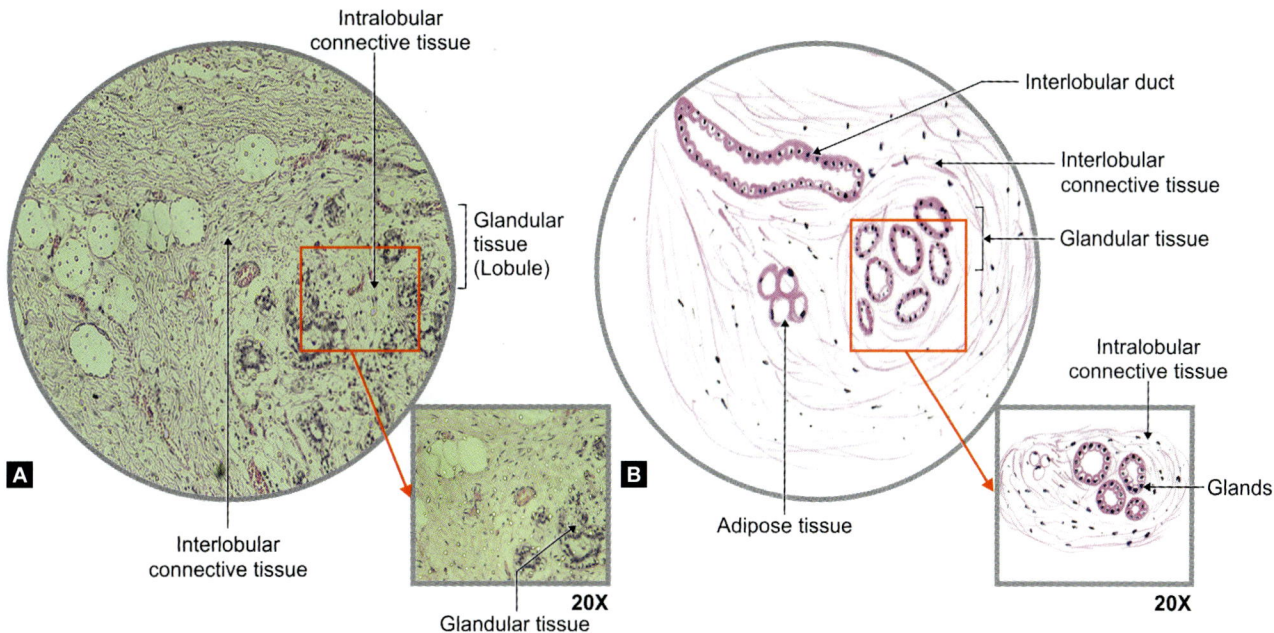

Figs 17.7A and B: (A) Microphotograph: Mammary gland (Inactive)(4X, 20X); (B) Diagrammatic representation

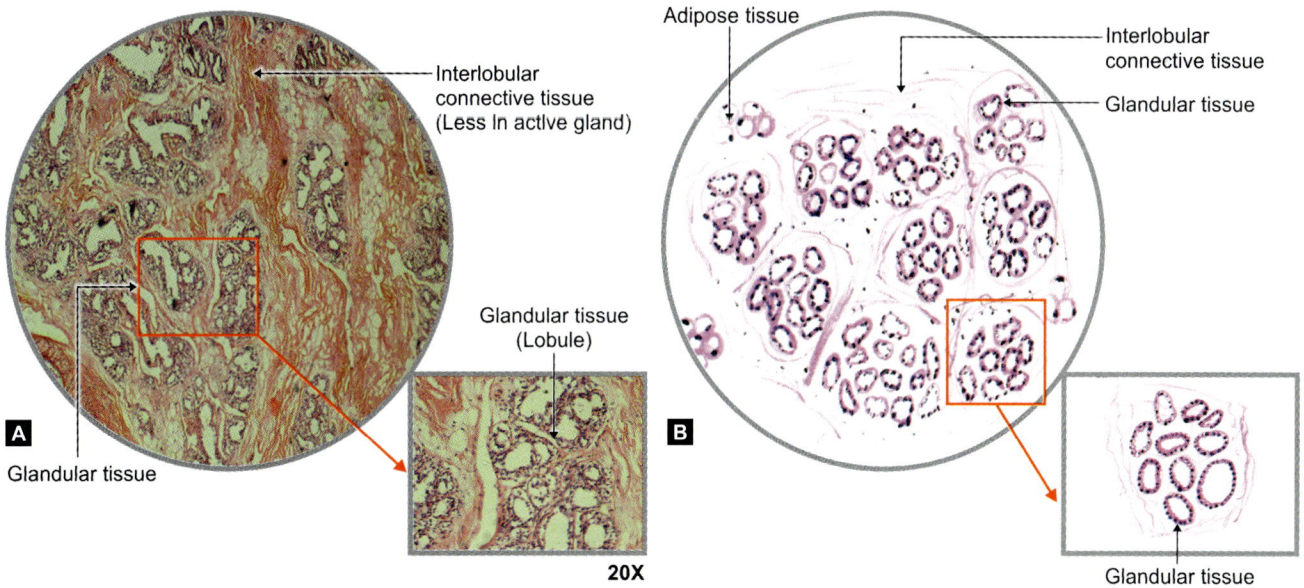

Figs 17.8A and B: (A) Microphotograph: Mammary gland (Active)(4X, 20X); (B) Diagrammatic representation

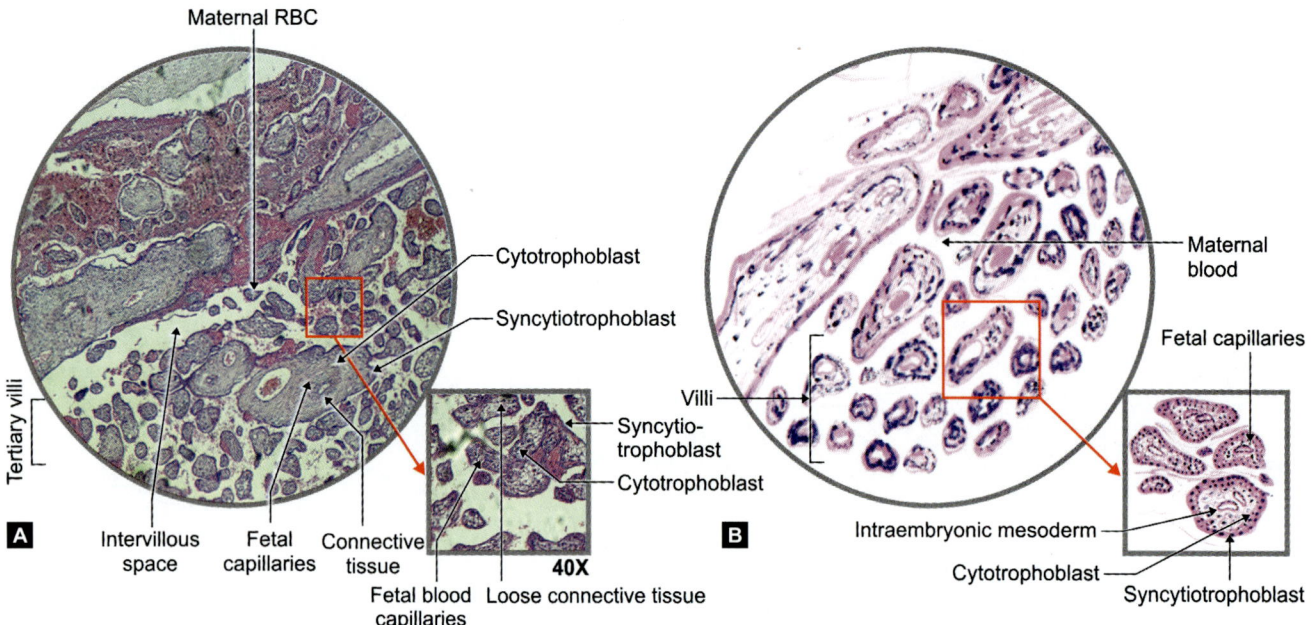

Figs 17.9A and B: (A) Microphotograph: Placenta (4X, 20X); (B) Diagrammatic representation

18 CHAPTER

Endocrine System

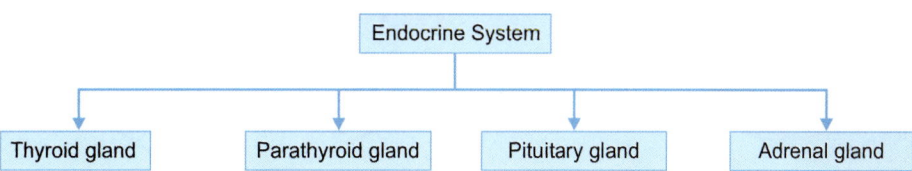

- Endocrine tissue is made up of cells that produce secretion which are poured directly into blood
- Secretions of endocrine glands are called hormones
- Highly vascular.

THYROID GLAND

- Covered with capsule
- Follicles with squamous to low cuboidal to columnar epithelium depending on functional status of gland. In the connective tissue there are parafollicular cells—secrete calcitonin.

PARATHYROID GLAND

Parathyroid chief cells (small, dark staining) and oxyphil cells (light staining).

PITUITARY GLAND

Consists of capsule and parenchyma
Adenohypophysis:
- Pars distalis
  - Chromophobes
    - Smallest cells (pale staining), in clusters
  - Chromophils
    - Acidophils-
      - Rounded cells- eosinophilic
      - Contain secretory granules- mammotrophs, somatotrophs
    - Basophils-
      - Polygonal cells-basophilic
      - Contains secretory granules- thyrotrophs, gonadotrophs, corticotrophs.
- Pars intermedia
  - Follicles filled with colloid substance
  - Lined by cuboidal cells
  - Produce MSH (melanocyte stimulating hormone).

Neurohypophysis:
- Unmyelinated nerve fibers and pituicytes
- Herring bodies are present.

ADRENAL GLAND

Cortex

- Zona glomerulosa
  - Ovoid clusters, curved columns
  - Cells- small (columnar to pyramidal) with round darkly stained nucleus

- A rich network of fenestrated capillaries
- Secrete mineralocorticoids
- Zona fasiculata
  - Polyhedral large cells arranged in long cords which are 1–2 cell thick
  - Pale staining nuclei (may be binucleate)
  - A rich network of fenestrated capillaries
  - Secrete glucocorticoids
- Zona reticularis
  - Small cells (Both dark and lightly stained)
  - Anastamosing cords
  - A rich network of fenestrated capillaries
  - Secrete DHEA, glucocorticoids

Medulla
Chromaffin cells- large, pale staining
Sinusoidal capillaries.

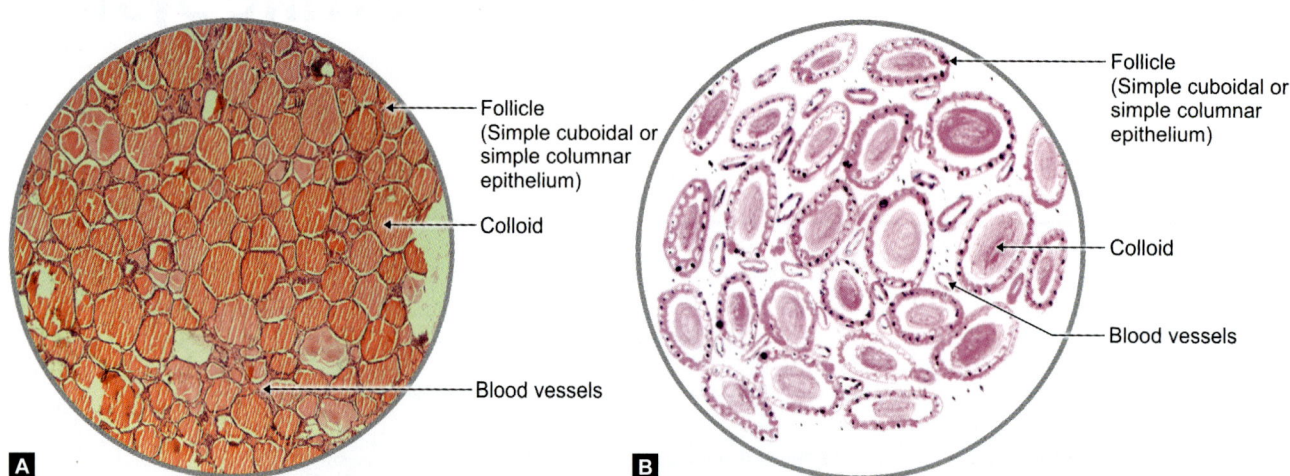

Figs 18.1A and B: (A) Microphotograph: Thyroid gland (4X); (B) Diagrammatic representation

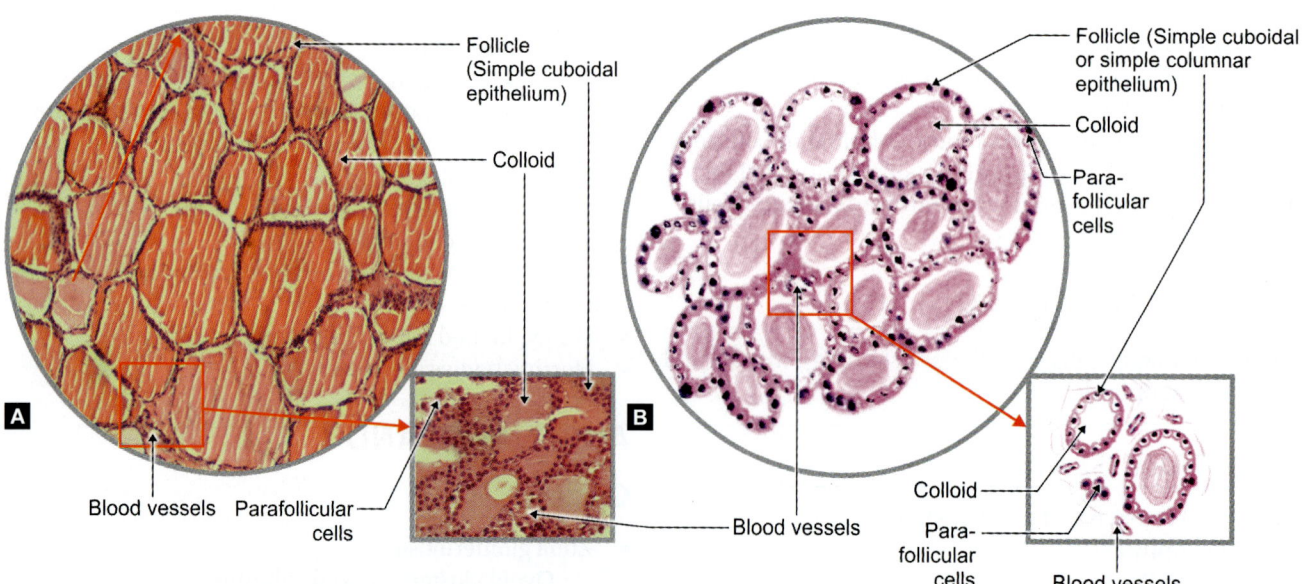

Figs 18.2A and B: (A) Microphotograph: Thyroid gland (20X); (B) Diagrammatic representation

Endocrine System

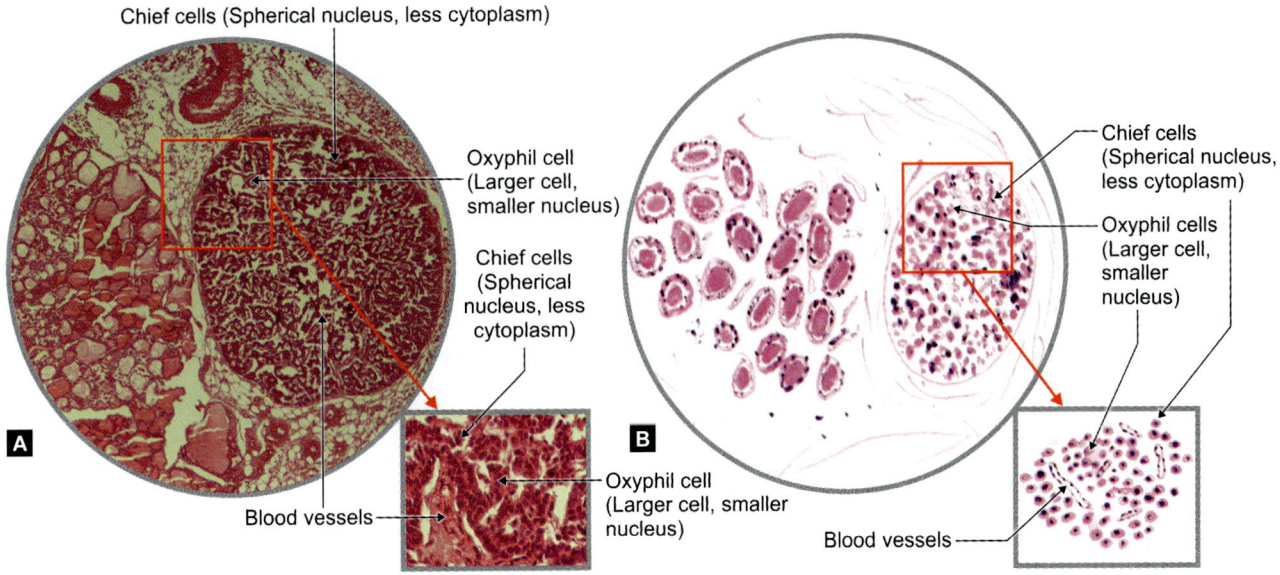

Figs 18.3A and B: (A) Microphotograph: Parathyroid gland (4X, 20X); (B) Diagrammatic representation

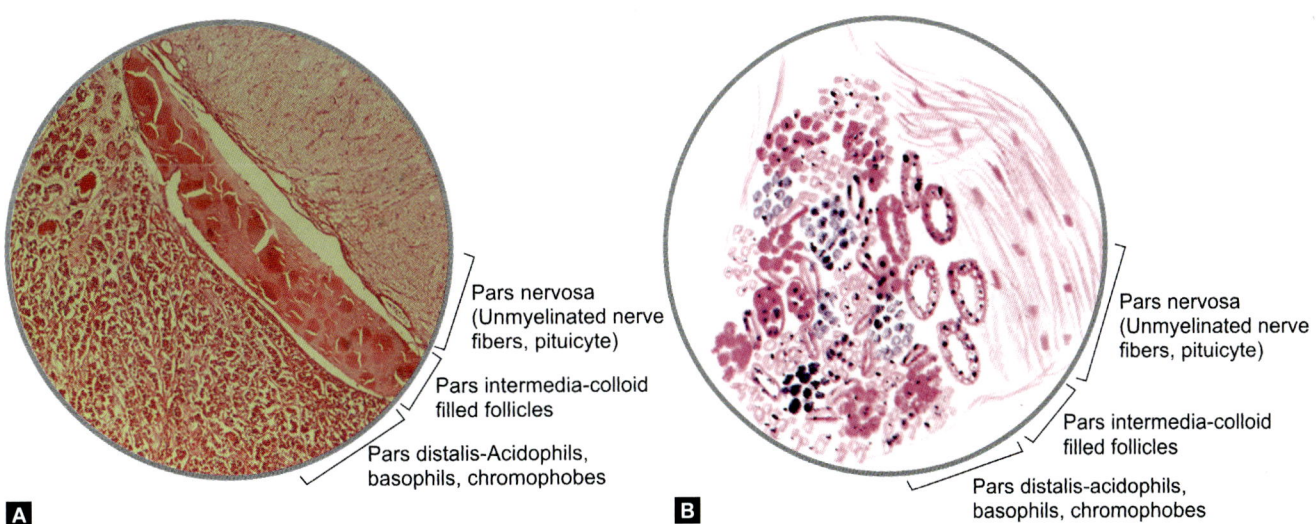

Figs 18.4A and B: (A) Microphotograph: Pituitary gland (4X); (B) Diagrammatic representation

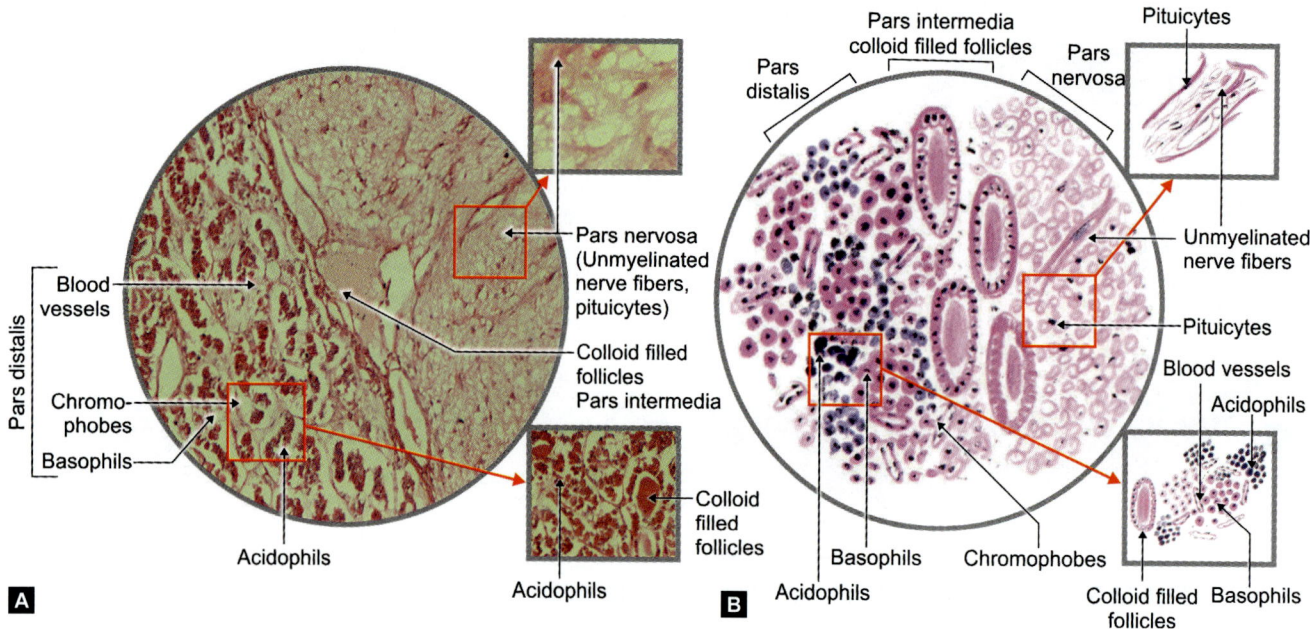

Figs 18.5A and B: (A) Microphotograph: Pituitary gland (20X); (B) Diagrammatic representation

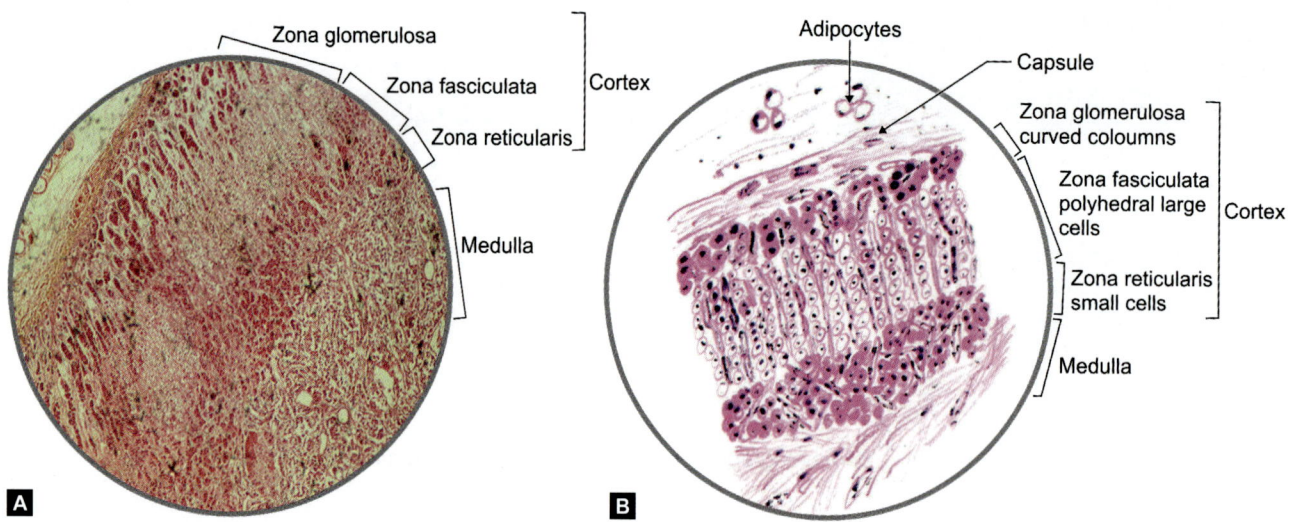

Figs 18.6A and B: (A) Microphotograph: Adrenal gland (4X); (B) Diagrammatic representation

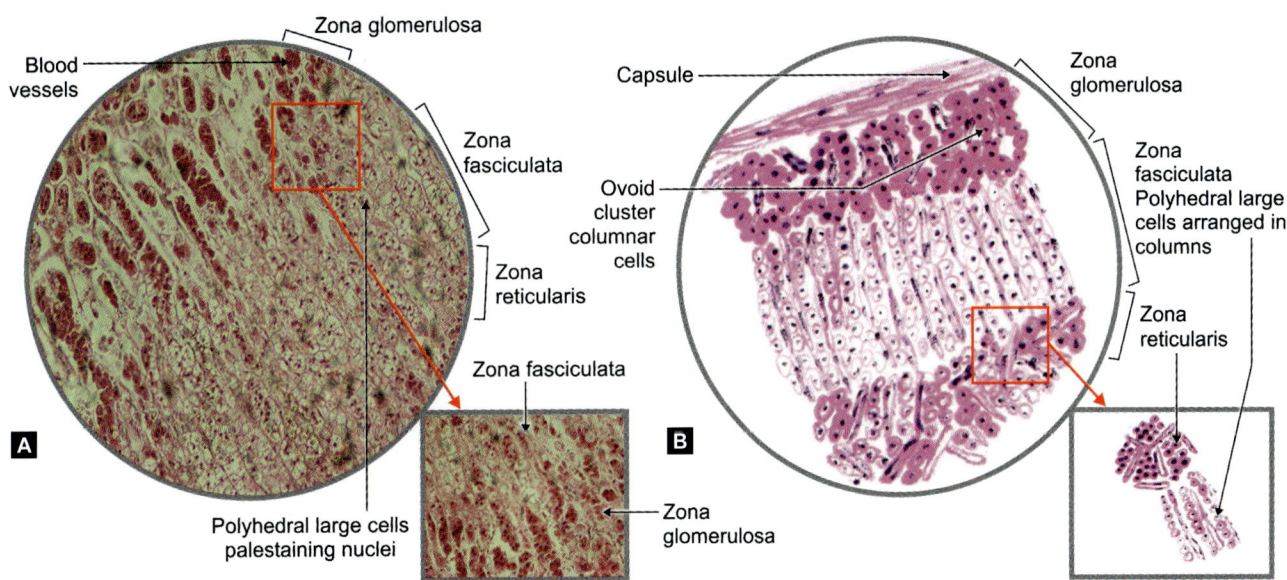

Figs 18.7A and B: (A) Microphotograph: Adrenal gland (20X); (B) Diagrammatic representation

19 CHAPTER

Eye

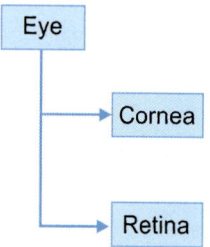

CORNEA

Thick transparent, nonvascular structure of eye.
Has five layers:
1. Epithelium stratified squamous nonkeratinized.
2. Anterior limiting membrane or Bowman's membrane (Collagen fibers).
3. Corneal stroma (substantia propria), collagen fibers and fibroblasts.
4. Posterior limiting membrane or Descemet's membrane (Collagen fibers).
5. Posterior epithelium simple squamous or cuboidal.

RETINA

Innermost coat of eyeball. Ten layers:
1. Pigment cell epithelium— cuboidal, melanin
2. Layer of rods and cones
3. Outer limiting membrane
4. Outer nuclear layer— nuclei of rods and cones
5. Outer plexiform layer
6. Inner nuclear layer
7. Inner plexiform layer
8. Layer of ganglion cells
9. Layer of optic nerve fibers
10. Inner limiting membrane.

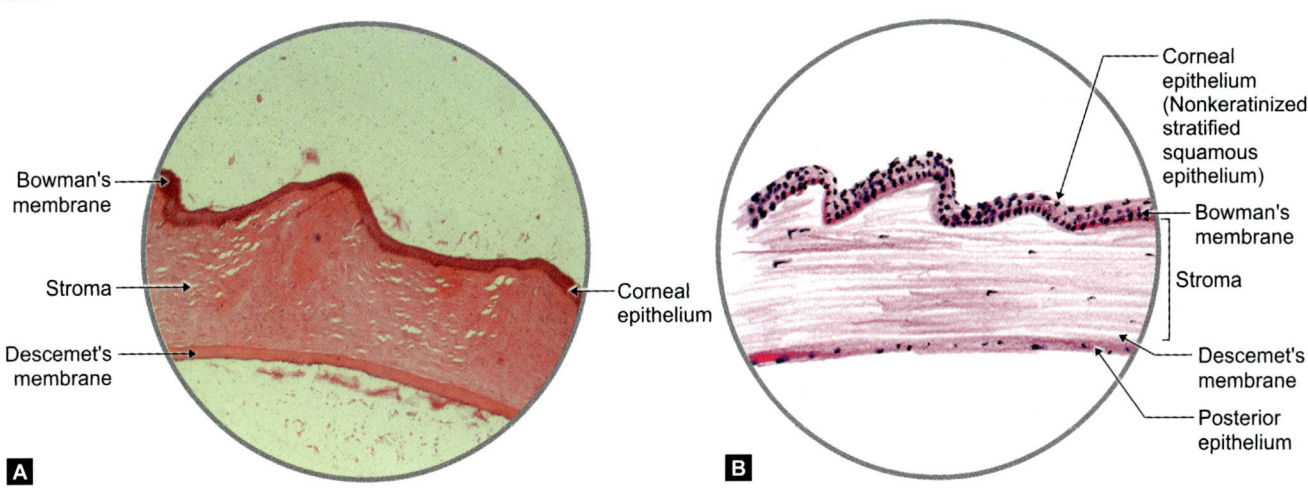

Figs 19.1A and B: (A) Microphotograph: Cornea (4X); (B) Diagrammatic representation

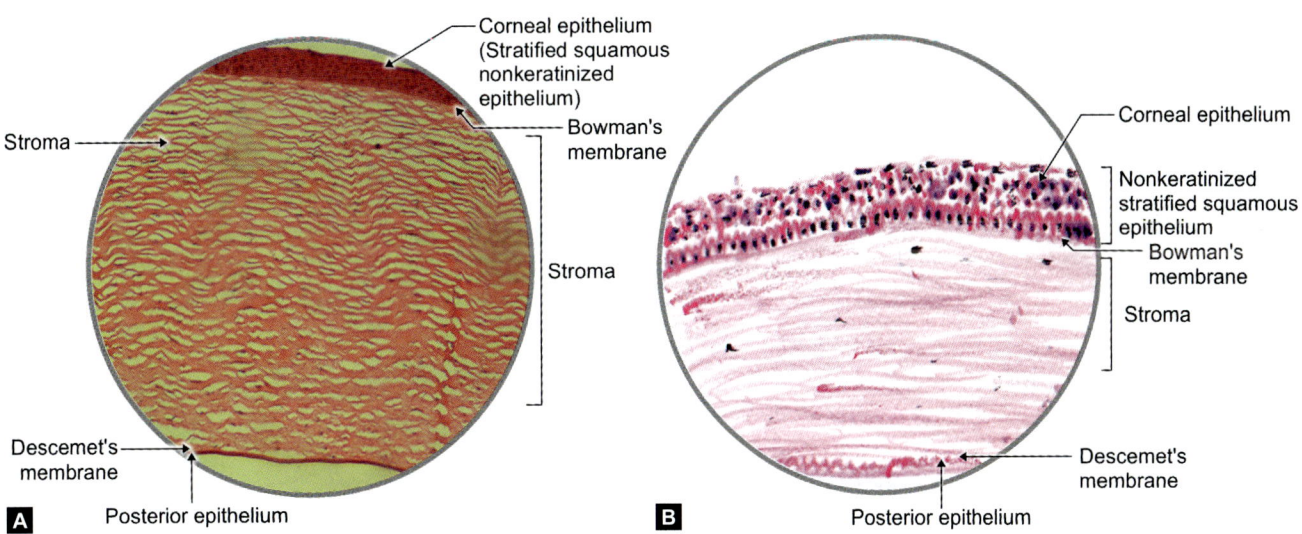

Figs 19.2A and B: (A) Microphotograph: Cornea (20X); (B) Diagrammatic representation

86 Atlas of Histology for Medical Students

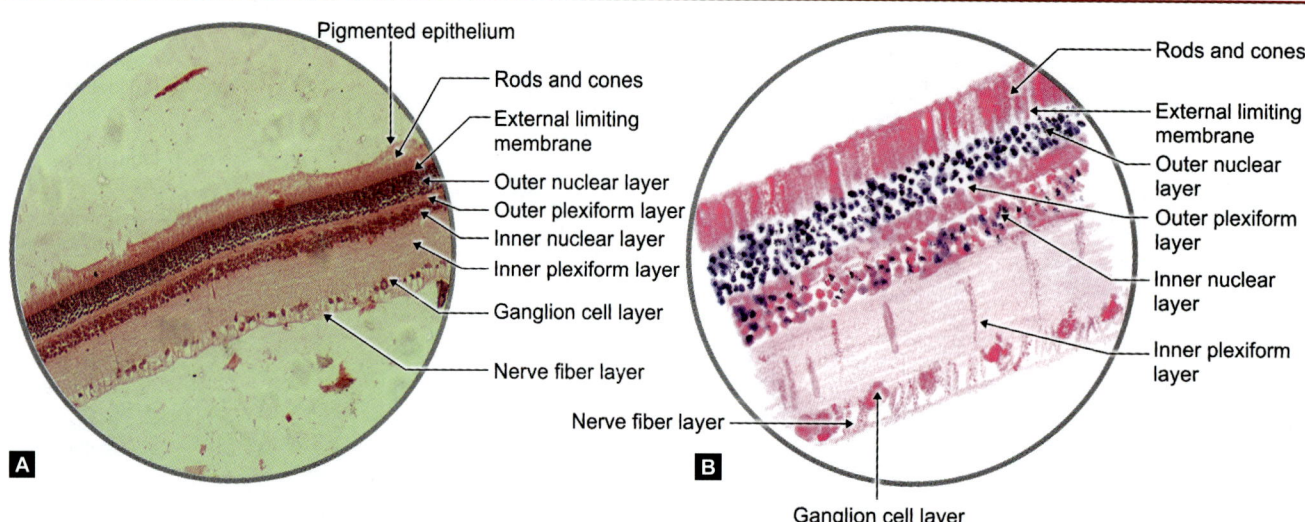

Figs 19.3A and B: (A) Microphotograph: Retina (4X); (B) Diagrammatic representation

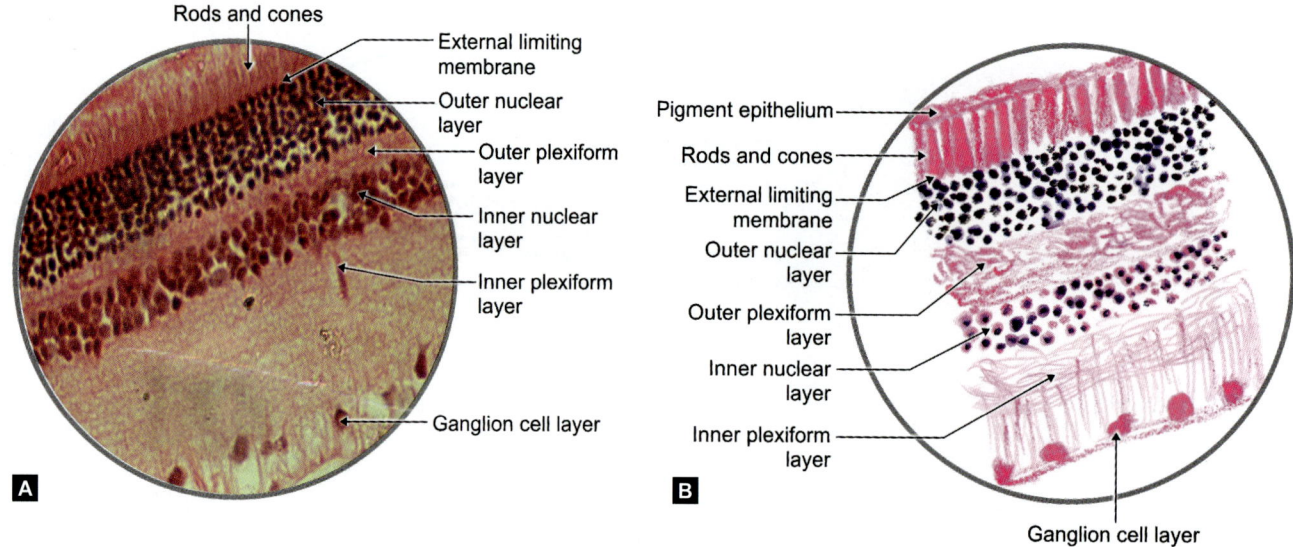

Figs 19.4A and B: (A) Microphotograph: Retina (20X); (B) Diagrammatic representation